NOON TO NIGHTFALL

To the Memory
of my brother Tony

NOON
TO
NIGHTFALL

♦

A Journey Through
Mid-life and Ageing

♦

by

Mary d'Apice

COLLINS DOVE
Melbourne Australia

Published by Collins Dove
A Division of HarperCollins*Publishers* (Australia) Pty. Ltd.
25-37 Huntingdale Road,
Burwood, Victoria 3125

First published 1989, reprinted 1990
Designed by Dimitrios Frangoulis
Cover design by Denise Korn
Cover Illustration Denise Korn

Typeset in Palatino 12½/13½ by Southern Cross Typesetting
Printed by Griffin Press Limited, Marion Road, Netley, South Australia

The National Library of Australia
Cataloguing-in-Publication Data:
d'Apice, Mary.
Noon to Nightfall, a journey through mid-life and ageing.
Bibliography
Includes Index
ISBN 0 85924 783 X
1. Middle Age. 2. Ageing. I. Title.
613'.0434

♦

Contents

Foreword

Noon to Nightfall is a timely book. In an age when the population of mid-life and ageing persons is increasing in most countries of the world, it is encouraging to hear the hopeful message which Mary d'Apice shares with us in her book. In the good company of noted scholars of human development, such as, Carl Jung, Bernice Neugarten, Erik Erikson and Carol Gilligan, Mary d'Apice has written an enlightening and useful book mapping out the journey through mid-life and beyond. Within a solid theoretical framework, the author breathes life into theory with well-chosen examples of flesh-and-blood adults who are negotiating these often perilous transitions with few, if any, road maps. Readers will find themselves resonating with Mary d'Apice's treatment of spirituality, anger, the ageing body, stress and burnout, sexuality, suffering and death, generativity and many other issues which shape the warp and woof of the mid-life and ageing process.

The field of adult development is relatively young. For almost one hundred years, we have had numerous resources charting the pathways of childhood and adolescent development, but it has been only in the last thirty to forty years that books and journals on the psychology of the adult life cycle have appeared on library shelves. Unlike childhood and adolescence where stages of growth and development follow more uniform lines, the movements that integrate adult life reveal greater diversity and uniqueness. While some adults follow what has been called the normative and expectable life cycle, many adult lives are not so neatly patterned. Later marriages, early deaths, unexpectable career shifts, and unanticipated divorces invite some to knit together a wholly different pattern. This book is important for two reasons: first, it offers a clarifying vocabulary to help us name our experiences more accurately, and second, it gives us an overall paradigm from which we can learn and against which we can test our own maturing identity. As Mary d'Apice says: 'To know something of the changes occurring during the second half of life empowers us to work toward wholeness and integrity.'

In addition to exploring the universal patterns of mid-life and ageing, Mary d'Apice also examines the fundamental differences between women and men as each matures through adulthood. Her treatment sheds new light on the recent findings in gender studies and helps the reader to discern and clarify the baffling conflicts that often emerge between and among the sexes during the second half of life. For many decades the norms for adult development were based primarily in the male experience. Most theories were conceived, articulated and written by men and then generalized to describe the whole population. Mary d'Apice has researched carefully the work of female developmental psychologists and has effectively nuanced the predominantly male theories with the feminine voice. Not only does this approach add to the understanding of the female experience of mid-life and ageing, but also it enables men and women to learn from one another's differences.

While the first half of life is concerned with themes of 'growing up', the second half addresses the agenda of 'growing down'. It is a time to engage in healthy introspection: to take stock, to reevaluate, and to challenge long-held assumptions and beliefs. This is the age when a woman experiences a new sense of autonomy and begins to imagine new possibilities for her post-parental life. And this is the time when a man often discovers the high emotional price he has paid for submerging his intimacy needs in order to compete and achieve in the work place. And for all, one's attitude towards ageing is an important factor. Victor Hugo had this in mind when he said 'forty is the old age of youth, fifty is the youth of old age.'

Carl Jung tells us that among all his patients beyond the age of thirty-five, every problem he heard could be related to a deep yearning within the person for a religious perspective on life. Jung was not speaking about organized religion as much as he was pointing out that in the second half of life, women and men begin to wrestle with meaning-of-life questions. There is a desire to make sense of one's life and to interpret one's life story within the larger story of the human community. Reassessing the meaning of love and work, and shaping a religious outlook on life are often the substance of the soul-searching that occurs in mid-life and the later years. It is to these timely issues that Mary d'Apice's *Noon to Nightfall* speaks with a most compelling voice.

James R. Zullo

Acknowledgements

There are many hundreds of men and women whose encouragement and enthusiasm have inspired me to write this book. I am grateful to these mid-life and more aged participants in seminars and workshops in various parts of the world. Their promptings were the reason I have undertaken this task and their generosity in sharing their own experiences has helped me understand more clearly the journey through life's afternoon. My gratitude is extended, too, to Jim Zullo of Loyola University of Chicago whose able presentation first opened up the fascination of this time of life, and I thank him also for his graciousness in consenting to provide the foreword to this book.

I should like to express my appreciation to all those Religious of the Sacred Heart who have shown their interest and backing in many different ways and to my Provincial for allowing me the time needed to complete this book. My special thanks goes to the members of my own community, Sisters Betty McMahon, Ethel Newman-Watt and Maria Vincent. Their unfailing support has helped over many a difficult moment. I am grateful also to Madeleine Wright representing the firm of publishers and to those who have added to the value of this book by their reading of the draft manuscripts and helpful suggestions offered: to Mary Anne Confoy, Nancy Kane, Phil Kilroy, Adrian Lyons, Bette Moore and Jim Moran. A debt of sincere gratitude is owed to Bert and Jean de Hosson for their generosity in making a word processor available for this work, and for continued interest in its progress. My thanks, too, to Sister Elizabeth Grantham for permission to use her unpublished poem 'Unless the Seed'.

But above all I am indebted to Sister Dorothy Ormesher without whom this book would never have been completed. Her unfailing assistance and encouragement, together with her skilful handling of the word processing and the hours of her time given so generously, have all been instrumental in bringing this work to a conclusion.

Mary d'Apice
Kerever Park, 1989

Chapter • 1

LIFE'S AFTERNOON

It happens every so often in life that we suddenly find ourselves living a dream which has been ours since childhood. So it was one January day when I found myself gazing up, in the crushing heat of midday, at a towering monolith in the heart of Central Australia. Ayers Rock glowed red in the heat of noon as the sun seemed to dance at its zenith — a powerful symbol of strength, courage and endurance.

Not many hours later, I stood silent with a group of tourists from every part of the world, watching in the hush of late afternoon as the rays of the setting sun played in a harmony of colour on the rock's smooth slopes. The beauty of evening, as day reluctantly let go its hold on the world, was reflected on the rock's surface and the massed clouds above in a kaleidoscope of changing hues. Finally, as we watched, filled with awe, deep violet melted gently into darkness. Night had fallen and even the birds were hushed into silence.

I thought of the changing beauty of the rockface from the sunlit splendour of midday to the calm serenity of evening. As I marvelled at the contrast brought about by the sun's passage from noon to nightfall, the words of Carl Jung came back to me: 'There is something sun-like within us.'[1] Our journey through life can well be compared with that of the sun as 'in the morning it arises from the nocturnal sea of unconsciousness and looks upon the wide, bright world which lies before it in an expanse that steadily widens the higher it climbs in the firmament. In this extension of its field of action caused by its own rising, the sun will discover its significance; it will see the attainment of the greatest possible height ... as its goal. In this conviction the sun pursues its unforeseen course to the zenith ... At the stroke of noon the descent begins. And the descent means the reversal of all the ideals and values that were cherished in the morning. The sun falls into contradiction with itself.'[2]

How many men and women have looked to the zenith, the noon, of their lives as the moment when they will have reached their goal, only to find that, once there, like the sun they seem to have 'fallen into contradiction' with themselves. It is only in the tranquillity of the evening that many reach a sense of fulfilment and of meaning that was not experienced in earlier years.

During the first thirty to forty years of life effort is very much centred on adapting to the surrounding world, 'the wide bright world which lies before us'. This known world makes many demands upon us. The person we become in the first half of life is one fashioned by these outside forces. As someone rightly said, we are named first by the world about us. It is not until the second half of life that we are able to name ourselves. True identity emerges from our own inner world and finds expression in the person we choose to become.

Too many miss this opportunity to become more authentically themselves through lack of understanding of the deep psychological and spiritual changes taking place in the early and late afternoon of life. The sense of confusion, weariness, restlessness or anxiety is so overwhelming that they abandon the inner journey and settle for a busy-ness which distracts from any further insearch. For others, the fear of the self they may discover paralyses their movement to wholeness. They are not free, and are left stunted and superficial in their approach to life, never really reaching full maturity.

To know something of the changes occurring during the second half of life empowers us to work towards wholeness and integrity. The known is under our control, the unknown so often poses a threat. Inner exploration, undertaken with some cognisance of what may be discovered, leads to a possession of oneself, to risking change and allowing transformation. It is this critical information that I hope this book will help to provide.

Life is a journey, a voyage to explore who, at depth, we really are. This entails not only a discovery, but requires also an integration of these newly found aspects of ourselves, a task that is not always easy. Like all travellers, we can find direction clearly only when supplied with a map to guide us through the various regions and possible obstacles ahead. Each will certainly take a different route to reach a uniquely personal destination, to become the person he or she has the hidden potential to be. Who then can supply an adequate ground plan covering so many various paths? Today's psychologists assure us that, in spite of the differences, there is a common underlying life-pattern that all must follow from childhood to their mature years.

Carl Jung speaks of four crucial changes to be undergone during the course of life — four times of breaking out of an existing pattern to emerge, even as a butterfly does from the chrysalis, into a new and unfamiliar world.

The first of these 'births', as he calls them, brings us face-to-face with a strange and threatening world as the security and safety of the womb is left behind. Few have ever stopped to think of what a momentous and traumatic change in their existence that must have been.

The second such rupture comes as the young person, now in the teen years, begins to break through the bonds of dependency on parents and home to become his or her own person. The emergence of sexual powers leads to the seeking of new relationships as the adolescent assumes responsibility for whatever the future holds.

It is at mid-life that we experience the third birth. Here we must negotiate the stormy waters of the transition from the first to the second half of life. We are faced with the discovery of our own inner world and the task of making this previously unconscious component part of the whole unique person we are becoming.

At the close of life, the evening time, the last birth or passage confronts each one. We let go our hold on life as we have known it, to be born into the unknown, uncharted territory beyond death.

Each of these new beginnings can well be compared with the metamorphosis which takes place when a caterpillar meets the uncertainty of change and spins about itself a web of thread. Have you ever wondered what takes place within the chrysalis before the emergence of a creature so entirely different from what it was before? How the thick body can become so slender, the stubby legs so long and graceful? Those who know speak of a complete disintegration before the re-formed body of the butterfly takes shape. Nature forces this delicate creature to emerge from cool darkness into bright sunlight and discover that the only option open is to spread new wings and to trust itself to the void.

During life many similar transformations are experienced, moments of re-birth, when we discover within powers and possibilities which up till that time had been hidden, unknown and undeveloped. Each such metamorphosis brings with it the darkness and pain of transition, but also the hope and joy of re-birth.

For many the most difficult of all these births comes as they cross the threshold of their 'second journey'. Jung maintains that the difficulty and possible suffering entailed prevent the majority of people from successfully passing through this transition. They shrink from the pain and loss which faces them. As one religious woman who was struggling in this crisis wrote: 'Sometimes I feel as though I'm in a cocoon, fighting my way to break the web and discover the new life that is waiting. Often I feel a bit anxious because I sense that the new life means letting go of the known, the practiced; and it doesn't happen that the new person emerges and the old just disappears. The struggle continues. But I think the eventual conversion cannot help but make a difference. It is extraordinary how difficult it is to accept myself and to be contented with the person God created and whom he loves.'

In the midst of chaos and upheaval something fresh is taking form, a new personality is struggling to be born. Grace is gently urging us to allow this transformation, to pass through the dying of the old to the new life beyond. For those who do successfully negotiate this passage, there lies ahead a time of new-found freedoms, fresh hopes and ripened maturity. New horizons open as deeper insights are gained into ourselves and others. We are no longer bound by the demands and expectations of the world around us but move gradually into the possession of our own deepest truths.

Mid-life, then, can be seen as an immensely important time, yet far too few people are aware of this. 'Worst of all,' Jung remarked, 'is that intelligent and cultivated people live their lives without even knowing the possibility of such transformations. Wholly unprepared, they embark on the second half of life.'[3] He goes on to ask where are the colleges and schools that teach us how to cope with the dramatic change which reverses so many of our ideals and truths; when 'what in the morning was true, will at evening have become a lie'. At the time of his writing, there was little opportunity for the ordinary man or woman to find any assistance in negotiating this transition.

In recent years, however, help has become far more readily available to those in their late thirties or early forties. Interest in this time of life is now well to the forefront of society. Our screens are flooded with films centred on the problems of mid-life, often humorous, sometimes more serious. Library shelves are rapidly filling with books on the handling of the crisis and the ensuing years. It has suddenly become fashionable to be middle-aged. Why this abrupt change?

Up until fairly recent years little research had centred on the changes taking place at this stage of life. This may have had something to do with the prolonging of the average life-span that has occurred over the past 150 years. Statistics reveal that, whereas in 1850 men and women had an average life expectancy of only forty years, by 1900 this had increased for men to forty-eight and for women to fifty-one. In 1970 women could look forward to seventy-four years and men sixty-seven years of life, whereas at present the life expectancy for women has increased to seventy-nine and for men to seventy-two. (Australian Bureau of Statistics).

When the life-span was shorter, the child at twelve or thirteen was initiated into adult ways, including preparation for marriage, leaving insufficient time for the freedoms of adolescence. The young adult, highly involved in the pursuit of work or in managing a family, moved quickly into the category of the aged. There was little or no mid-life span for the majority of people. The marked increase in life expectancy means that women now can look forward to almost as many years of life after the end of their child-bearing years as before. People in the workplace can expect ten or more years of retirement. This necessitates a serious re-adjustment in the lives of most. A clearly defined period of adult development between the late thirties and mature or old age is now widely recognised.

In the last few decades, many psychologists have been drawn into a study of this period, carrying out research in the world's leading universities. Some compare the changes at mid-life with those occurring in the identity crisis of adolescence and go so far as to speak of middlescence. However there is at least one considerable difference in the two stages. We are, at forty, far more able to take control of what is happening: to act, as it were, as co-creators with God in this work of growth and second flowering. The task of naming ourselves has commenced and the person we become will, from now on, be very much our own responsibility.

What is it, then, that underlies these changes taking place in the transition from young adulthood to middle-life? There would seem to be five major causes to be recognised. The first could well be described as a sociological one. Social institutions, such as industry, government and religion, which shape and mould our lives, make slight allowance for the changing needs of this stage of development. Present day society has not yet caught up with the altering patterns of life. To those young adults who, in their thirties, have 'made it to the top' and have nowhere else to go, it offers little incentive for venturing into new ways. It gives scant support at this bewildering time of change. A sense of frustration, boredom or unease begins to creep in where previously job satisfaction was high. For many, this may be the first step leading to the crisis of mid-life.

An hormonal imbalance also begins in the mid to late thirties as the reproductive powers of both men and women start to decline. This can result in marked emotional instability. The effect of an imbalance in the opposite direction during adolescence is readily recognised, yet we tend to forget that this reversal also plays its part in many of the 'problems' faced at mid-life.

In addition, as already hinted at, deep psychological changes underlie much of our altered approach to life. The movement into an inner world reveals many unknown areas of our personality. This can be a confusing, and even traumatic, experience before we gradually perceive the potential hidden there. So fascinating is this alteration in the human psyche that the next few chapters will be spent in exploring it at depth.

Both men and women can, too, be far more affected by the physical diminishments — or increases! — taking place in the early forties than they are sometimes willing to admit. Much of mid-life grieving may centre around the physical losses they experience at this stage.

The final underlying cause of the transition taking place is a powerful spiritual transformation. This occurs gradually with the passage through the unrest of crisis to a new level of maturity. A deep conversion is frequently the outcome of the struggles we undergo and the pain we experience at this time. 'We are not converted once in our lives,' Thomas Merton wrote to a friend, 'but many times, and this endless series of large and small conversions, inner revolutions, leads to our transformation into Christ.'[4]

Faced with the awareness of these determinants many people try to avoid or deny them, seeking to hold on to what has served them well in the past, whether it be in values, dress or behaviour. They try to put the clock back, often with unfortunate results. Others recognise and welcome the change and modify and re-arrange the circumstances of their lives to allow for wider interests or the development of new creative powers. For some, this second journey will entail a completely new direction. One professional man chose at forty-five to leave his medical career and to take up cabinet-making with remarkable success. Others find a new energy for and dedication to the way of life they have already chosen, committing themselves more deeply to its fulfilment.

There is a beauty and a challenge in these years which is often overlooked. Mid-life can be the most exciting and important time of life. If we have the courage to embark with hope on this journey into afternoon, the adventure will bring with it untold rewards. What at first appeared as contradiction will show itself as a new truth, the source of fresh ideals and values. The pain of re-birth will gradually give way to the joy of a deep acceptance of oneself. It is a time of growth, of integration and of becoming more fully the unique person each was destined to be.

The self-possession born of a satisfactory negotiation of these years sows the seeds of a serenity and peace which intensifies and deepens with the passage through the later years. The evening of life then becomes a time of continued involvement and enrichment, while the older person gradually readies him- or herself for the final separation.

♦ ♦ ♦

Chapter • 2

EXPLORING UNIVERSAL PATTERNS

Underlying every life there is a hidden universal pattern despite the unique circumstances and conditions in which that life is lived. All tend to follow a similar, though apparently different, path as the life cycle unfolds. Psychologists have gradually become aware of this design, especially in the past sixty years, and have described it in various ways as they seek to highlight one or other aspect. It can be confusing for the uninitiated to find so many seemingly differing descriptions of the stages of development. But diverse as these appear, they are not conflicting and, once understood, can add a richness and a new dimension to our lives. Let us look then at some of the best known of these theories, those of Jung, Erikson, Gilligan and Levinson.

Carl Jung, a Swiss psychiatrist, was born in the Thurgau Canton in 1875 and died in 1961 at his home in Zurich. He is generally acclaimed the 'spiritual father of the life cycle theory'. Sigmund Freud, his close friend and colleague for many years, could not agree with many of the developmental changes recognised by Jung. This, among other differences, finally led to the break up of their friendship just before the First World War. Jung was thirty-eight years of age at the time, and it was perhaps the loss of this relationship that plunged him into what today we would call a severe mid-life crisis. Using his own experiences and those of his patients as his major source of information, he continued his research alone. In case this might have been seen to prejudice his findings, Jung wrote in one passage: 'Most of my patients are socially well-adapted individuals, often of outstanding ability ... one-third are suffering ... from the senselessness and aimlessness of their lives.'[1]

From these he recognised the four crucial changes or births, already mentioned. Two of these he saw as belonging to the first phase of life; one started at the meridian or noon of life and the final one occurred for most at the conclusion of life's afternoon. He was quick to stress that although there were two distinct phases in life as he described it, the second was in no way less important than the first. 'The afternoon of life is just as full of meaning as the morning; only, its meaning and purpose are different.'[2]

At the heart of Jung's psychology lies his recognition of the importance of the unconscious and its function in our lives. It is from there that this change of meaning and purpose derives. Only a small proportion of our psyche is conscious in earlier years and this gradually increases. It is especially in the second half of life that a more rapid expansion of consciousness occurs, and much previously unconscious material emerges. The psyche can be compared to a massive iceberg whose tip only appears above the surface of the ocean. The bulk which lies below is what can threaten shipwreck to the unwary. One of the tasks at mid-life is to have the courage to explore this previously unknown part of the personality.

Jung speaks of this unconscious part of the psyche as a combination of our own personal unconscious and what he calls the collective unconscious. The former is made up of all those experiences which for various reasons have been forgotten, repressed or barely recognised in consciousness. The latter consists of contents which 'have never been in consciousness and, therefore, have never been individually acquired, but owe their existence exclusively to heredity'.[3] The recognition of this area of the unconscious came as a revelation to Jung and was confirmed time and time again through the study of his patients and of the myths and fairy-tales handed down through the years. 'I can only gaze with wonder and awe at the depths and heights of our psychic nature,'[4] he was once to say.

He described the collective unconscious as made up essentially of archetypes, 'inborn and universally present formal elements'[5] or patterns which embody typical situations in life. Jung spoke of these as having 'form but no content'[6], and in 1936 wrote: 'Archetypes are like riverbeds which dry up when the water deserts them, but which it can find again at any time. An archetype is like an old watercourse along which the water of life has flowed for centuries, digging a deep channel for itself. The longer it has flowed in this channel, the more likely it is that sooner or later the water will return to its old bed.'[7] It is the content of the archetype, the water so to speak, that each provides from his or her own individual experience of life.

What Jung is saying here is that all typical experiences, situations or unlearned modes of behaviour are archetypes to which we react with a typical response. Examples of some of the archetypes he identified are the great mother, death, the wise old man or woman, the shadow, the journey of the hero and a host of others. These arise from the inherited collective unconscious and are filled with their distinctive content from each one's personal unconscious. Thus the archetype of the 'great mother' will be coloured by our own experiences of being mothered; the anima (see page 53) will in some way reflect the women in our lives. In a dream Geoff, in his mid-forties, found himself lost in a labyrinth of long, dark tunnels, and filled with fear of the dangers he felt lurking in the darkness. A woman suddenly appeared beside him and taking him by the hand led him through the maze to the opening of the tunnel. There lay a wide sunlit meadow. Coming into the light he found his guide to be a gentle fair-haired young woman, 'in every way the image' of his sister. This meeting with one aspect of his anima encouraged him to welcome his own gentler feminine side.

Jung saw archetypes as patterns in the psyche which in a way are analogous to the instincts in the body. They provide meaning and direction in the journey of individuation, of reaching one's unique wholeness. This concept of archetypes may be difficult to grasp at first. It will, hopefully, become clearer as we examine the task of encountering and integrating some of them, in chapter 4 of this book.

In his autobiography, *Memories, Dreams, Reflections,* Jung describes two distinct personalities: one belonging to life's morning and formed in response to the people, events and institutions of our environment; the other, the result of the meeting with our inner world, an encounter with the previously unconscious, in the second half of life.

Young children only gradually begin to dissociate themselves from those around them, especially from

De Colores!

Chris Boerner #230

I am so happy you are working this Cursillo weekend! Bless your heart for sharing your time and talent, and for serving in this way.

I want you to know that in the week preceding this weekend, I listened closely to the messages from the Christian radio station, KTIS, and offered up these "learnings" in your name. I also turned off the heat each time I drove my car, in order to focus my thoughts on you and the beautiful meaning behind Cursillo!

Arise, Come to your God

Turn Your Eyes Upon Jesus

Amigos De Cristo

He is the Bread of Life

parents or carers, and become aware of the 'I'-ness that is theirs. The first half of life is spent developing this conscious personality centred on the ego which, in Jungian terminology, is the centre of the awareness of individuality: myself as myself. The person I begin to know as myself is the one shown to me by those around me, and the image I hold of myself will depend on what others think of me. It is they who name me in this first stage of life. How many are the people we have met who, by the time they reach mid-life, are consumed with a real hatred of the person they perceive themselves to be, through the constant messages they have received. 'I feel I am nothing more than garbage,' one client said. She was the neglected child of an alcoholic father. To alter this attitude can become one of the most difficult tasks of mid-life, but necessary for growth to full potential. Each of us has a responsibility to help others to see themselves as worthwhile, since, especially in early years, a sense of self-esteem depends so much on the affirmation of those around us. I shall ever be grateful for the change in my life resulting from a simple affirming remark about the way I once read a passage of poetry.

It is those about us also who influence us to choose the aspects which become part of our conscious personality. The possibilities of the opposites, which are also within us, are banished temporarily to the unconscious. It is these whose re-appearance so often surprises and even disgusts us in the second half of life.

Another of the tasks in life's morning is to develop a persona or mask through which one relates to the outer world in a way acceptable to it and satisfying to oneself. Each develops a number of these public images according to need. So the doctor presents one mask, his or her professional persona, to deal with patients, another on returning home as partner or parent. A healthy persona, as John Welch points out, is one which fits the expectations I have of myself, those which others have of me and is also true to the reality of my personality.[8] Without this grounding in my own personality the persona becomes a trap from which I find myself unable to escape. Many religious people have put such stress on others', or their own, expectations of what a priest or religious should be, that their persona is no longer true to their own personality. They tend then to identify with their role, to become the 'good sister' or the 'devoted brother'. One woman owned that she had become trapped into two roles, that of principal of a school and the wife she thought she was expected to be. No longer did she know who she really was herself, nor could she give expression to the deep feelings which were an essential part of her personality.

The consolidation of the first and conscious personality, is usually completed by the time mid-life is reached. The ego is then central, giving a strong sense of identity and purpose. It is with dismay that we discover a second personality emerging, one which challenges our established attitudes and ideals.

The work of individuation, as Jung saw it, has now begun. The change taking place in the orientation from the outer world to the inner, and the resulting development of the second personality, was so significant in his eyes that he used the term individuation to describe this process of differentiation, which leads to becoming one's own self. 'We could,' he tells us, 'translate individuation . . . as "self-realisation."'[9] Jung did not deny that individuation starts much earlier in life but stressed that it was only after mid-life that the process assumed its true significance. It is then that the imbalance between the many opposites in the personality strives for equilibrium.

One revelation of these opposites comes to us through the emerging archetypes, especially those of the shadow and the animus or anima (see chapter 4). Finally the Self, the archetype of wholeness, assumes the central role previously held by the ego.

The Self lies dormant in earlier life, deep within the unconscious, while the ego is accepted as central to who we know ourselves to be. Only as we pass into the second half of life does the true Self, like the sun, begin to rise to consciousness and we find that our world, like that of Copernicus, is in its rightful place only when it is orbiting around this sun.

The strong emphasis on interiority, the movement to explore the inner world, adopted by Jung is not as evident in the well-known theory of Erik Erikson, a German by birth, who completed most of his research in the USA. A sociologist and historian as well as a psychoanalyst, he introduced aspects of all these disciplines into his understanding of development. The basic attitudes he described as central to each of his stages of development, were a combination of inward experiences, observable behaviour and unconscious inner states.[10] His stress on the influence of culture and relationships on the development of both the child and the adult is of particular interest and was first outlined in *Childhood and Society* in 1950. In a chapter entitled 'The Eight Ages of Man' he elaborated his understanding of psychosocial development, as it occurred from the child's earliest years until the adult reached old age. As the chapter heading indicates, he is writing here of male development. Although he did recognise a difference in the sequence of developmental stages in the two sexes, he did not incorporate any change into his schema of the life cycle. It was Carol Gilligan who was to demonstrate this difference most clearly nearly thirty years later (see page 25).

Erikson's theory rests on the identification of eight psychological strengths or qualities, the development of which indicates that the individual is ready and able to cope with 'the structure of the social institutions'[11] which he or she is meeting at various times in life. These strengths are in potential, in seed as it were, within the psyche from birth, but mature fully only when the circumstances of life call them forth. Something similar might be seen in the case of a garden planted with a variety of seeds and bulbs. Each will start to grow only when the climate and conditions are right for it, and it is itself ready for such growth. Some seeds will lie dormant until winter, while others will have produced flowers in the spring or fruits in autumn. Others, such as the desert-oak or the waratah, may need a major catastrophe, a bushfire, to awaken the life within..

Erikson recognised a certain sequence in the growth of these qualities and of their becoming the focal issue at each critical period of development. This, for the most part, was dependent on external life structures. The need of the infant for nurturing, of the child for play and the older adolescent for career are some of the factors responsible for stimulating the growth of these strengths. As the individual encounters each new significant situation he or she is faced with two contrary dispositions, one he called syntonic, the other dystonic. (See figure 2.1). The satisfactory emergence of the new strength will depend on the balance achieved between these two impulses. Erikson speaks of these self-confrontations as crises or turning points in life. They are not usually accompanied by a serious emotional disturbance, though this may sometimes be the case. As a result of each of these crucial periods

Figure 2.1

Psychosocial stages of life

Old age								Integrity vs. despair WISDOM
Adulthood							Generativity vs. self-absorption CARE	
Young Adulthood						Intimacy vs. isolation LOVE		
Adolescence					Identity vs. confusion FIDELITY			
School age				Industry vs. inferiority COMPETENCE				
Play age			Initiative vs. guilt PURPOSE					
Early childhood		Autonomy vs. shame, doubt, WILL						
Infancy	Basic trust vs. basic mistrust HOPE							

Source: Erik H. Erikson, Joan M. Erikson & Helen Q. Kivnick, *Vital Involvement in Old Age*, W.W. Norton & Company, New York, 1986, p.36

individuals find themselves in some way different and, hopefully, better fitted for the task in hand.

The first and critical phase of development occurs in infancy. The infant, completely dependent on others for food and care, is faced with the impulse to either trust (syntonic) or mistrust (dystonic) the mother or custodian to meet its needs. Which of these attitudes dominates will depend largely on the baby's carer. For the child whose basic needs are wisely satisfied in answer to its cries, a sense of trust will become strong. The neglected child will develop an equally strong sense of mistrust in those around it. The infant who is cared for in such a way that trust can develop naturally will form a basis upon which hope can be fostered and will grow. Hope is the first of the psychological strengths to appear as the result of this interaction between the self and the world. It is essential to human existence. Without it life cannot be sustained, as has been found in many orphanages where abandoned children have lost all hope, and with it, life. This hope is the basis of our ongoing faith throughout life, a confidence and belief not only in others, but also in ourselves and above all in God.

The optimal climate for the development of any of the psychological strengths is one in which there is an integration which blends both syntonic and dystonic elements, with the syntonic dominant. Maldevelopment can result from a disproportionate emphasis on either element. In the case of the infant, the constant fulfilment of its slightest whim will lead to over-dependence, a certain naïveté, and an inability to tolerate any disappointment in later life. Insufficient care will lead not only to lack of trust, with subsequent difficulties in relating, but may give rise to a complete withdrawal from others. The mother or carer can err in either direction with a resultant hindrance to the healthy development of hope in the child.

There is, however, opportunity for this, or any of the other stages, to be re-worked later on in life. Maladaption as the result of too much of the syntonic element, in this case trust, can be re-worked later in life either spontaneously or with the help of a therapist. It is a more radical task to correct an overemphasis on the dystonic, mistrust.

Many become aware in their middle years that their relationship with others or with God is one of fear rather than trust, and that hope is dead in their lives. Such an awareness can constitute the initial movement towards the re-integration of this basic level. For this to happen, it is necessary that they find someone whom they can risk trusting in at least one area, perhaps a spiritual director, counsellor or therapist. With some stable support, they can be encouraged to gradually move out in trust to others. One woman portrayed this dramatic change in her life in a series of sketches. In her early pictures she showed herself without any recognisable facial features. The final drawing showed a smiling face with eyes shining. Under it was the hope-filled caption: 'It is good to be alive!' At last she had dared to trust another and in doing so had found new life.

I have elaborated Erikson's first stage of development more fully in order to give a better understanding of his theory. The following stages of childhood and adolescence will be dealt with only briefly, while those of adulthood and mature age will be amplified in a later chapter.

As the two- to four-year-old gains in strength, the possession of greater self-reliance becomes evident. It is faced then with the choice of relying on its own power and developing a sense of autonomy, or being filled with doubt and shame. Developing sphincter control is an important area in which the child begins to experience his or her autonomous power to hold on or to let go, to be in command. The encouragement of the mother in careful toilet training or in allowing adequate freedom for the toddler will strengthen the syntonic impulse. This will allow for the growth of the psychological strength of will or self-determination. The sense of justice acquired in later years will rest on that foundation.

In play the young child is able to develop the sense of initiative, to be inventive in games using imagination freely. Provided this remains within limits which respect the rights of others there will be no sense of wrong-doing. When initiative outweighs guilt it gives rise to purpose, the psychological strength of the play age.

Schooling should rightly encourage competence or skill in the young person on the basis of a healthy balance between the attitudes of industry and inferiority. This will be critical for the child's self-esteem now and in the future. Unfortunately, lack of encouragement from teachers and/or sometimes parents, too often leads to a pervasive sense of failure which remains throughout life or until the stage can be reworked later. Constant correction or punishment in childhood has resulted in a sense of worthlessness in many adolescents.

As childhood is left behind the adolescent faces decisions for the future, for career and also for relationships. Failure to find employment or a meaningful friendship on leaving school frequently leaves the young person unsure of his or her identity. For boys, the sense of identity has traditionally been closely linked with the choice of career, for girls it has been associated more with that of relationships. Recent research confirms this, with the young women interviewed by Carol Gilligan defining their identity 'in a context of relationship and judged by a standard of responsibility and care';[12] the young men speaking rather of 'great ideas and distinctive activity'[13] in the descriptions of themselves. She proposes a reason for this as will be seen later in this chapter. As Erikson describes this stage, fidelity, the 'ability to sustain loyalties',[14] emerges from the resolution of the tension between the sense of identity and the inevitable identity confusion.

The attraction towards intimacy with another develops strongly in the young adult. At the same time there is a pull to remain apart, to isolation or solitude, for fear that the newfound identity be threatened by too close a contact. This may be true for men, but, as Erikson and others realise, it is in an intimate relationship that the young woman finds her true identity. For her, the stages of identity and intimacy are fused. From the correctly balanced tension between a desire for intimacy and a pull to isolation grows the first adult strength, love, a mutual devotedness which gives the capacity for a close and lasting relationship despite inevitable dissensions.

The movement into mid-life brings with it a deepening concern for all one has produced in life whether it be children, institutions or ideas. Erikson calls this quality care and sees it as the product of a crisis, in which generativity predominates over the dystonic self-absorption or stagnation. The person who can put aside self-interest for the good of others is the caring, generative adult.

In the final stage, as the ageing adult struggles to accept the 'inalterability of the past and the unknowability of the future',[15] to find integrity despite a pervasive sense of despair, the last great strength of wisdom becomes central. It is this which enables us to recognise the integrity of experience, the meaning of life in the face of death. 'I would not want to change my life in any way,' commented one eighty-year-old, in spite of years of suffering and of loss.

Erikson speaks of these stages as being epigenetic, each growing out of and building on the foundations of the preceding one. Not only does the successful handling of any stage depend on the satisfactory resolution of the earlier ones, but each movement forward requires a modification of the previous strengths to fit them for the current life situation. The autonomy reached by the three-year-old will need to be adapted to an autonomy suited to the school-age child or the self-determination appropriate to the ageing person. Similarly, the identity discovered at eighteen will undergo radical change with the movement into the middle years, and again as old age is faced. At each stage we are striving to develop not only the appropriate psychological strength but also to re-work or to modify strengths already gained.

Erikson's stages are not hierarchical in the sense that one is better or higher than another as is the case in Piaget's understanding of cognitive growth or Kohlberg's of moral development. They are interpenetrating, each in some way present in the current stage which predominates. While the person at mid-life is involved in an effort to become generative, at the same time he or she is re-working identity, and perhaps a level of trust and a new way of showing initiative and independence. The dignity which comes with the integrity of old age, is also slowly being acquired.

Erikson admitted that his scheme of psychosocial development was drawn from his observations of men and boys and that he was aware of the fact that women's progress through these stages was not as clearcut. The adolescent girl, he believes, holds her sense of identity in abeyance, often combining the tasks of identity, intimacy and generativity. A coherent sense of self may emerge only in a relationship of intimacy, where 'she comes to know herself as she is known'.[16]

Carol Gilligan, a co-worker of Kohlberg at Harvard University, took Erikson to task in 1982 in her book *In a Different Voice*. What she pointed out was that Erikson's model used as normative in development a process of separation, once the relationship of trust was established. This is the case for the growing male child who must learn to see himself as different from the predominantly female carers in the early years of life. The little girl, on the other hand, comes to identify with her carers and to model her growth on them. There must then, according to Gilligan, be a basic difference in the mode of development in the two sexes. To take as the norm a psychological schema of separation suited to the male, without introducing a corresponding model of attachment for women seemed to be a denial of the equality, though difference, in the development of women.

The difference in the psychology of women and men is repeatedly seen in the normal course of life. Nancy Chodorow argues that girls emerge from the earlier developmental periods 'with a basis for empathy built into their primary definition of self which boys do not'.[17] The play of children, a major sphere of socialisation, gives further evidence of divergence in orientation. Janet Lever[18] observed that girls tend to play less competitive games than do their counterparts, in smaller, more intimate groups and are less concerned with rules than they are with the maintenance of relationships.

At adolescence, whereas the boy finds his identity or coherent sense of self in relation to the world and his career, giving rise to further differentiation and separation; for the girl, the experience of identity is fused with that of attachment. For her, intimacy and identity are intricately interwoven. In a close relationship with another person she comes to know herself most truly, and is inclined to be fearful of separation, while the young male can find intimacy threatening.

The strength of care in a woman which develops strongly in the years preceding mid-life extends not only to her children but also to the adults in her world. Women's strong point, her concern with relationships, is often, as Jean Baker Miller observes,[19] considered by men in early adulthood as a weakness rather than a human strength. The discovery by men in their mid years of the richness of intimacy, relationships and care is something women have been aware of all along. Their development through this to equal maturity with the opposite sex has not yet, however, been explored in an area of research which has, in the past, been dominated by men.

In proposing these basic differences in orientation between the two sexes Gilligan did not address in any way the theme of the boy's attachment and identification with the father-figure in his life or the little girl's need to differentiate herself from the father-figure. As Fowler points out,[20] there can be no true picture of the development of women or of men without consideration of these factors. This is yet to be done.

The importance of relationships and the responsibility of caring they involve is also seen by Gilligan to be at the root of the difference in men's and women's moral development. Kohlberg's stages of moral development, based on research with men, accepts as its goal the acquisition of the universal principles of justice and rights. For women, however, the final goal of moral development, according to Gilligan, is to obtain a mature attitude of responsible care for both oneself and others, a focus on the dynamics of interrelatedness rather than justice. This by its very nature precludes violence and harm either to others or to oneself. 'Thus the logic underlying an ethic of care is a psychological logic of relationships, which contrasts with the formal logic of fairness that informs the justice approach.'[21]

One woman seemed to move to this final stage of morality during the course of a seminar on mid-life development. On the morning of the second day she had a story she wanted all to hear. The previous evening on her return home she had found her twenty-year-old son and his girl friend obviously awaiting her arrival. She was tired after a long day of concentration so sat down with them in the lounge. After 'failing to notice' his twice repeated suggestion that she might get the dinner, she was relieved to see that it had finally occurred to both young people that they might do it for her. This was the first time in her married life that she had ever considered her own needs (in this case for rest) as equal to those of others. For her, 'the good or the right' had been to serve and provide for her family, no matter the cost to herself. Now she realised that 'the better thing' was to recognise the interdependence of her own legitimate needs and those of others. There was no need to do violence to herself. Such was her delight at this change in her perception that she could not wait to share the excitement of this new discovery.

The 'different voice' with which women speak tells of a basic dissimilarity in the way they and men relate to the world. It is to be hoped that the effect this has on their development will one day be more fully researched. The separation theme which characterises male development from early childhood until mid-life contrasts with the attachment theme which runs through the whole life journey of women. 'Their embeddedness in lives of relationship, their orientation to interdependence, their subordination of achievement to care'[22] leave them, according to Gilligan, with a different truth to that of men. As she asserts so strongly: 'Only when life cycle theorists divide their attention and begin to live with women as they have lived with men will their vision encompass the experience of both sexes and their theories become correspondingly more fertile.'[23]

In the first and the final chapter of his book, *Seasons of a Man's Life,* Daniel Levinson sincerely regrets this lack of direct concern with the female life cycle and development in general.[24] Although the original group for his research included women, financial pressures made it necessary to restrict the final sample to forty men from four different occupational settings. However, I have found, as have others, that, in spite of the basic differences in outlook, women relate closely to the structure he describes. It is for the reader to agree or disagree.

Levinson commenced his research into adult development at Yale University in 1968 and published his results just ten years later in the book referred to above. Although he relied heavily for his understanding of adult development on both Jung and Erikson, his approach differed from theirs. He was concerned rather with the search for a life structure, some universal patterning or sequence, which, while allowing for cultural and individual variations, would be a constant in all lives. He discovered this in the identification of four distinct eras or seasons, each lasting approximately twenty to twenty-five years and separated from the preceding one by an introductory transition period, or crisis, of four to five years. None of these seasons he saw as richer or more important than the others. Yet each was as different as winter — a fallow time of preparation for new growth — is from the springtime of fresh green shoots or the full-blown flowers of summer.

Developmental periods in early and middle adulthood

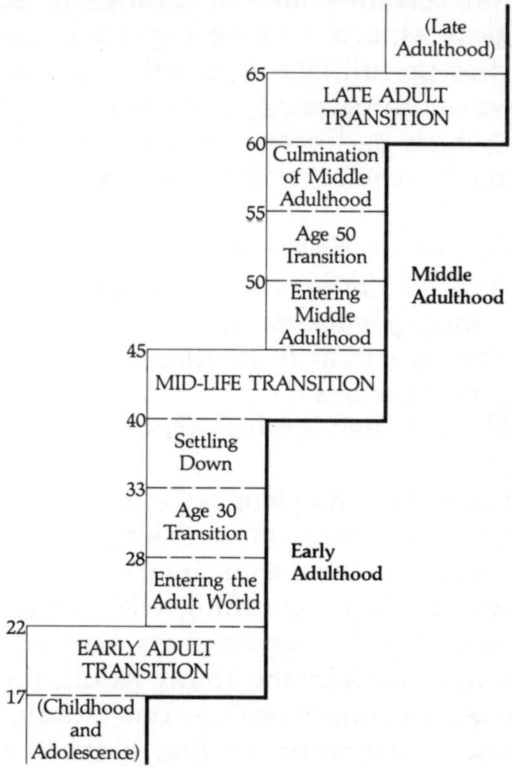

Source: Daniel Levinson *et al.*, *The Seasons of a Man's Life*, Alfred Knopf, New York, 1978, p.57.

Figure 2.2

These eras, including the transition periods, correspond to the years of Childhood and Adolescence up to seventeen, Early Adulthood from seventeen to approximately forty, Middle Adulthood up to sixty or sixty-five, followed by Late Adulthood (See Figure 2.2). Each season has its own special beauty, its time of blossoming and of producing its distinctive fruit. The transition periods are those times in which the basic character of life belonging to an era is modified and changed in preparation for entry into the new season. They are occasions of crucial change in life. Within each season certain common biological, social and psychological aspects can be expected, and certain tasks need to be fulfilled if growth is to continue.

There was nothing particularly startling about this discovery which had been known in a less scientific way for many years. As Shakespeare once told us:

All the world's a stage
And all the men and women
merely players ...
And one man in his time plays
many parts,
His acts being seven ages ...[25]

What did surprise and delight Levinson and his co-workers were the clear-cut divisions in each of the eras. He found that the men he interviewed showed an astonishingly regular patterning within each season. The period of roughly seven years after an inter-era transition, whether it be the Young Adult, the Mid-life or the Late Adult transition, was one of adjustment to the new social structures of life, a fairly calm and stable period of development. This, in each case studied, was followed by a period of about five years of re-evaluation, of possible structure-changing — a transition within the era. This was not usually as severe as the re-orientation of the inter-era transitions, which proved to be the major turning points in life. Another period of stability followed each of these mid-era transitions before the men moved into the transition heralding the next of life's seasons. This pattern of alternating periods of stable development and transitional structure-changing was evident in each of the subjects studied and was closely linked with age, though not age-specific. A degree of variation existed according to psychological, social and biological readiness and conditions.

In the language of the playwrights, Levinson's structure could well be described as a play in four acts, his seasons, each dealing with a different facet of life's journey. As in a Shakespearean drama, each act is separated from the next by an intermission, one of the major transition periods, while the scenes within the act deal with a similar theme and are demarcated by a less noticeable interlude, or transition.

In exploring Levinson's scheme of the adult life-structure, we find the young man or woman in the early twenties emerging from the Young Adult transition into a period of life which Levinson names Entering the Adult World. This is the time, in the twenties, when careers — or the preparation for them — and sometimes life partners, are examined and chosen as the young adult begins to build a stable life structure. The passage into the Age Thirty transition gives rise to a period of restlessness and dissatisfaction towards the end of the decade. For many this transition brings a deep uncertainty and a painful sense of doubt as to the wisdom of the choices made earlier. This time of questioning interests or relationships and general unrest is followed by what Levinson describes as the Settling Down Phase in the early thirties. The emphasis here is not only on 'finding a niche' for oneself in society but also on striving to reach the top of one's career or profession. Some speak of this as the 'ladder period'. Levinson also calls the last few years before forty the time of Becoming One's Own Man, with the appropriate acronym, as Leavitt points out, of BOOM.[26] Women, whether or not they are in the work force, appear to experience a similar striving for fulfilment at this period of life. For them, however, this resides more in connectedness, interdependence and care than in separation and differentiation as it tends to in men.

The Mid-life transition, commencing in men at about forty or earlier and in women usually at about thirty-six, starts for many with the sense of falling from the ladder. The echoes of the BOOM fade away in the distance and we are faced with the slump. If the middle years bring with them a marked alteration in activities of caring or in relationships, this will deeply affect the mid-life woman.

As we stand on the threshold of this new season we are acutely aware of the lack of support offered by society and the paucity of possible role models to be found for this stage of life. The questions which confront the majority at the mid-point of their journey are: 'What have I done with my life?' 'Have the values I hold been lived out as I would have liked?' The answers to those questions, as we penetrate our inner world and meet so many areas previously denied, is usually in the negative. There is a sense of uselessness, even of repugnance as stock is taken of earlier years. This time of disillusion and depression has been spoken of by some authors as a 'creative illness' because it is frequently the forerunner of new purpose, energy and enterprise.

Levinson's next phase is that of Entering Middle Adulthood where the task is one of modifying the life-structure. The Mid-life transition has been a time of searching and re-evaluation. Now life must be so re-organised that it can be enriched by the many new possibilities which are opening up, the altered outlooks or new values and perceptions. Untried enterprises may beckon or creative pursuits entice. A fresh vitality and vibrant involvement in living is often seen in the late forties.

At about age fifty a time of crisis or transition, with all the struggle involved, is once more encountered. It is not uncommon for this to be experienced as deeply disturbing, more so possibly than the one heralding mid-life. If, for some reason, a person at forty has been too preoccupied to allow a true experience of the mid-life transition, this may catch up with him or her in the early fifties. The deep disorientation and unrest experienced then enables the re-structuring missed out earlier to take place.

The concluding years of the third season in life, called by Levinson Culmination of Middle Adulthood, can be years of rich fulfilment and stability. George Vaillant emphasises that this can also be a time when a crisis not mentioned by Erikson, can be encountered. He speaks of the struggle between keeping the meaning and rigidity. Vaillant sees this in some way fitting in between the crises of generativity versus stagnation and integrity versus despair. There is a temptation to hold on to things as they have been rather than to see that the old meaning or tradition can still survive well in different modes of expression. Perhaps one reason for this is the regret that our generation is declining, our personal control lessening. A new age is beginning to take over. As one man summed it up: 'I get upset when I see the younger generation ignoring the guidelines we lived by, but I suppose the future is in their hands as it was once in ours. They'll probably make a go of it just as we did.' These years in the late fifties are a quieter, calmer and more contented period of life than were the forties.

With the movement from Middle Adulthood to Late Adulthood, another transitional period is faced, not unlike those that have preceded it. Realising that retirement is close, a man or woman may be confronted by a real sense of decline and of fear of the future. This time of restructuring leads to a major turning point in the life cycle, a time of radical change in life-style. The birth pangs of this new season may be severe for some and hardly noticed by others.

Levinson's investigations have not, as yet, progressed further than this last transition. We can only conclude that a pattern similar to that of the earlier seasons will be followed throughout Mature Adulthood with a succession of more relaxed periods interspersed with times of greater pressure and struggle, especially as the diminishments of ageing are faced. These are years for reconciliation, a coming to a sense of inner peace with self and with the world.

The final years of life, those beyond eighty-five, are referred to as Late Late Adulthood. Levinson sees the continuation of development at this end period of the life cycle as coming to terms with the process of dying and a preparation for death. At the same time there is need to remain as far as possible involved in life, a model of 'wisdom and personal nobility'.[27]

Having explored what these four life-cycle theorists have to say about the patterning of life, we may well ask ourselves the question: 'How does the understanding of these theories help us in the working out of our own lives? How do they fit together to give a clearer description of our journey?'

Each of the theorists we have looked at is trying to examine one of the many and complex aspects of the normal growth to psychological wholeness. As Jung describes the sun's passage from the horizon to the meridian with its outlook on the world 'steadily

A synthesis of development theories

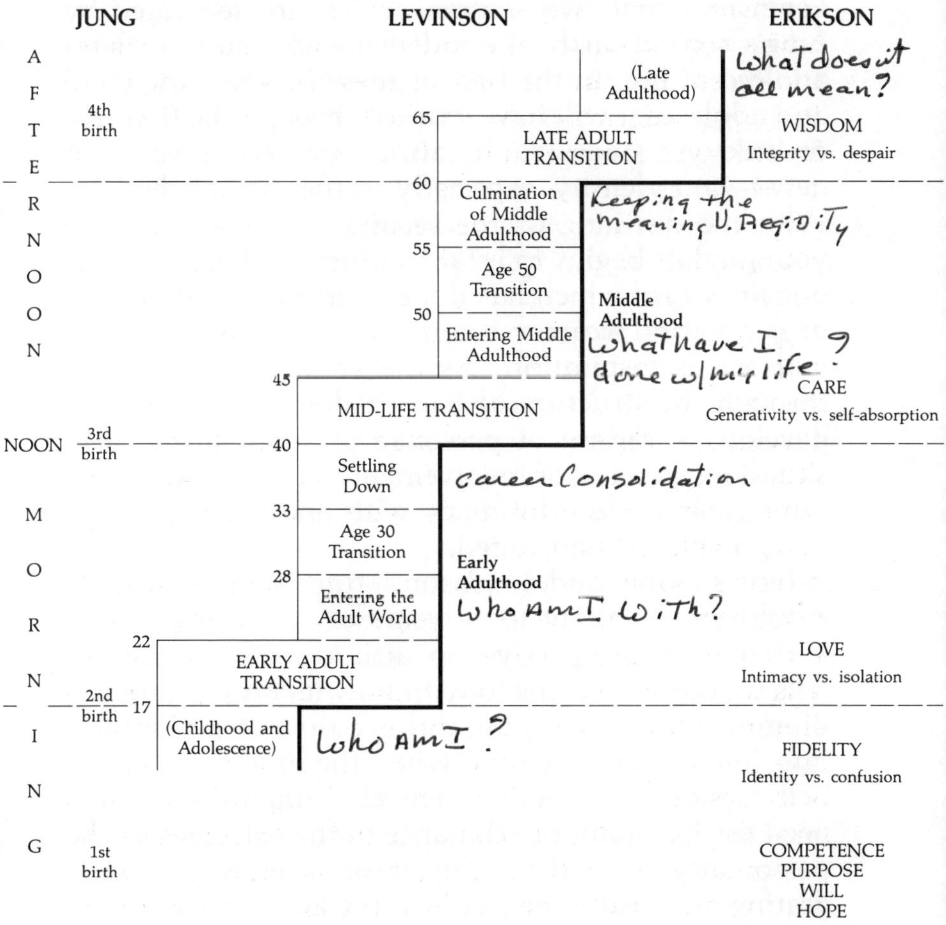

Source: Based on Daniel Levinson *et al.*, *The Seasons of a Man's Life*, Alfred Knopf, New York, 1978, p.57 and the author's interpretations of Jung and Erikson.

Figure 2.3

widening the higher it climbs in the firmament', we recognise the impact of that world on ourselves during the first half of life. This period embraces Levinson's first two seasons which are separated by Jung's second birth, the independence found in later adolescent life. In the first of these seasons, the child and adolescent will have worked through the first five of Erikson's stages culminating in a certain sense of new-found identity, especially in the case of the boy. With the dawning of the second era or season, the young adult begins to establish him- or herself in the outside world which has done so much to mould him or her, to find a career, a companion and a goal which will act as inspiration. As the young person moves through the structure of Early Adulthood, he or she develops a variety of personae to adapt to the new situations in a life of involvement with society. At the same time a closer intimacy with another is perhaps being explored and tested.

Jung's noon and Levinson's transition to Middle Adulthood at about forty years of age, brings about a change in perspective, in attitude. As the former tells us 'the sun begins to withdraw its rays in order to illumine itself'.[28] For Jung this is a time of exploration into inner depths, a time when the archetype of the Self is slowly becoming central, bringing with it a need for harmony or rebalance in the extremes of the personality. It is the moment of meeting and integrating more fully the shadow, the animus and anima and the neglected psychological powers. This, too, is stressed by Levinson as he speaks of the main task of mid-life as being one of bringing four major polarities into balance, of restructuring our lives, of forming new attitudes. It is during this stage that one struggles, too, with the need to be generative, to enrich the lives of others, and the inclination to self-absorption or stagnation. For many who have perhaps developed well in the area of generativity, a strong sense of identity may break through for the first time at mid-life.

All stress the importance of individuation in the second half of life where, Jung tells us, we are able to know ourselves, not only as the world has shown us but rather as our own depths have revealed. Levinson speaks of a freedom from outside pressures and expectations, a time of being 'less tyrannised by the ambitions, instinctual drives and illusions of youth ... The Self acquires an importance for a man roughly equal to that of the external world'.[29]

Levinson's stress is on providing an age-linked structure within which we see the tasks of life unfolding. Jung's is on exploration into the origin and integration of the psychological changes taking place both in early and later life. Erikson describes the phases entailed in the development of psychosocial strengths, from the moment we first put our trust in someone outside ourselves to the 'involved disinvolvement'[30] implied in the wisdom of old age. Gilligan attempts to bring to these theories an understanding of a theme of development different from that of separation, a recognition that ongoing attachments can be an alternate and equally valid path to maturity and self-actualisation.

♦ ♦ ♦

Chapter • 3

ADULT CRISES OR TRANSITIONS

When *Dante Alighieri* prefaced his First Canto of the *Divine Comedy*, the Inferno, with the words 'Midway upon the journey of our life, I found myself in a dark wood, where the right way was lost',[1] he spoke not so much of a physical journey but of the deep psychological changes which threw him into a state of confusion and terror at the noontime of life. His is one of the many and beautiful descriptions of this painful passage that all must traverse on the quest for wholeness. Another comes in a letter received after one mid-life seminar: 'Ten years ago I was a hopelessly self-pitying, self-centred, anxious person, settling for the pity of others because I could not imagine I was loveable. Now, because of my "creative illness" many of your words ring true in my life. Each day is an exciting gift, beauty in so many places and people, overwhelming joy and unbelievable strength. I can now face life.' This fifty-year-old mother of three had suffered a severe mid-life crisis and had found new life and hope as a result.

To appreciate what is taking place during these times of transition, it is necessary to understand what is meant by crisis. Crises, the dictionary states, are not only turning points or decisive moments but also times of acute danger or suspense. The Chinese have chosen to combine two ideographs, those for opportunity and for risk, to convey the concept of crisis. The Greeks use a word which expresses a searching or sifting through of information to come to a judgement. All these elements are caught up in some way in the crises known as developmental transitions. They are times of re-evaluation, of acknowledging the features of the preceding period, and of exploring new alternatives. When this work of re-organisation is completed we are ready to move into a new phase of life.

The resolution of crisis comes with the commitment to what has been judged best for the future, perhaps a new life-structure, perhaps a re-adherence to one already chosen. If this decision is undertaken too soon, before time has been allowed for the necessary space or maturity to consider all the options fully, one is said to foreclose. As a result there is an inability to live fully the new way of life and to find one's identity within it. Too early a marriage or the dedication to religious life without sufficient consideration will lead to such foreclosure, resulting in an identification with the role rather than a living-out of personal identity within it.

This has been the case often in the past when religious life was chosen at the relatively early age of thirteen or fourteen, before the young person was sufficiently mature to make a considered choice. As one brother confessed: 'It was only when I got into bed the night of my reception and saw a habit hanging on the door, that the choice I had made, or rather, what I had walked into without much thought at all, suddenly dawned on me.' The consequences of this lack of full decision could be a moulding into the externals of the life without any real ability to be freely oneself. The concern then is on what seems to be the appropriate way of acting or speaking, rather than on the expression of the true personality. The young man mentioned above, however, later opted strongly to continue in religious life and is still happily living out his vocation. The changes which have taken place recently in religious orders make this lack of true commitment far less likely to occur.

If there is no commitment, no personal investment, there is a tendency to drift from one thing to another, without ever being deeply involved in anything. We have all met these drifters. Today they can be highly enthusiastic about a new pursuit; by tomorrow they have tired of it. They move on elsewhere, always searching for something they never find.

The passage through crisis or transition needs to be rooted in a genuine seeking for a life-structure appropriate to the coming period of development. A gradual but sure adoption of this should then follow.

It is generally agreed that developmental crises may begin so subtly that we are often unaware of what is taking place. There may be nothing more than a sense of dissatisfaction; or restlessness or boredom may be the only indication. At other times these transitions seem to be triggered by an obvious occurrence, moving house, losing a job or the death of a loved one. A minister wrote of the shock of adjusting to a new parish at the age of forty. 'The move so jolted me that I wondered if I could possibly recover.' This change was the starting point of his mid-life crisis. Although many happenings in life are critical, especially loss through death, they are not all associated with the pattern of development. Only some may activate a developmental transition.

All crises are, however, experienced somewhat similarly. The difference lies in the fact that developmental crises or transitions lead to growth and, in spite of the confusion and trauma felt, are in the end energising and life-giving. Some of the critical periods in life, those that Erikson refers to as 'imposed, traumatic and neurotic crises',[2] are draining of energy. They lead to disintegration rather than to integration of the personality. It is often only in hindsight, as the Whiteheads point out,[3] that we are able to recognise the difference between these two types.

The onset of crisis can, therefore, be abrupt or imperceptible depending often on the causal factor. The way it is handled will depend very much on whether or not it has been anticipated or foreseen. To expect an event is to be prepared for it, and to be better able to survive it. That is one reason why Levinson's patterning of the transitions in life can prove so helpful. To know that times of disorientation and confusion are normal, alleviates much of the fear and concern often accompanying these periods of disruption.

The experience of crisis is described by some as a time of being confined in a dark tunnel. Or again, others feel carried in the trough of a wave with the constant threat of the crest crashing down upon them. However we image this ordeal, it is one characterised by a sense of loss, though what has been lost may not be apparent. At mid-life this may well be the passing of youth and its aspirations; as we approach our later years the deprivation of independence or the threat to an accustomed life-style may be the reality mourned. We need time to accept and grieve for this loss, before we can integrate it and proceed with our development.

The disorientation which accompanies the experience of crisis can sap the powers of concentration or the ability to 'stay with' someone. This is seen even in the eyes of many people in crisis. Their attention is constantly wandering and they seem to be in some distant world.

Not only is there mental confusion but the emotional disturbance is frequently more marked. A common vicissitude is the swing between the desire for others and the alienation from them, the need to be close to friends and the pull to isolation, to hide away in a corner. 'I can't even think of somewhere far enough away to escape from it all,' said one mid-lifer. The same confusion of feeling is present in our relationship with God, whom at times we long for in our loneliness and who seems at other times strangely absent and unwanted.

This fluctuation of feeling can be disconcerting to those wishing to accompany another through the time of crisis, unless they understand fully what is happening. The knowledge that a friend is always waiting in the background is the greatest support that can be given to anyone suffering emotional upheaval. It was Tagore, I think, who once said: 'There is rain in your soul, my friend, and I have no umbrella. But let me walk beside you for a while.' Quiet re-assurance is all that is looked for and is the best gift we can give.

Deep depression is often an accompaniment of crisis, as is a general lack of energy and drive. This gives rise to a fall-off in production. Work suffers and in spite of increased efforts success seems unattainable. There is a tendency to blame others for the situation, not through malice, but simply because we can no longer take the responsibility for failure.

The depth of pain and confusion is a healthy sign rather than one to be feared. It speaks of an openness to change, to growth, to integration. Those who laughingly speak of never having had to undergo such an upheaval may well be the poorer for this. Some may not have had the courage to face the crumbling of the world they felt was so secure. They shrink away from it, being unwilling to relinquish what has been precious to them up till now. These never know the enrichment that can come as a result of such disintegration.

Evelyn and James Whitehead, in discussing the structure of adult crisis, point to the fact that it is an opportunity of special openness to the action of God, a sacred or *kairos* time. It is 'in the disorientation of a crisis that the believer can experience the inbreaking of God, who challenges conventional insights and plans; in the journey through and beyond the pain of a crisis the believer can experience the grace of deliverance, the gift of being empowered to live a new and better life'.[4] There is usually little 'felt presence' of God in the midst of struggle and it is only in faith that we recognise his action.

The mid-life crisis

Now that my ladder is gone,
I must lie down where all ladders
start.
In the foul rag and bone shop of
the heart.[5]

W.B. Yeats in his poem, 'Circus Animals' Desertion', provides a very apt description of the crisis met by most in their late thirties or early forties. This most heralded and best known of all transitions has been the subject of countless poems, films, plays and novels in the past two to three decades. It has become fashionable to be forty, and acceptable to experience the collapse which so often characterises the noon of life.

The moment is reached when we must come to terms with what indeed does seem to be 'a foul rag and bone shop' as we look within. What brought with it so much satisfaction in earlier life, now seems tasteless, meaningless and without purpose, a tremendous waste of time. What was experienced as success, as reaching the top, has turned to ashes, and disillusionment predominates as the shift to interiority brings with it so much that seems negative and unwanted.

The crisis of the limits, as the mid-life transition is often called, puts us in touch with our own limitedness, apparent failures, and the seeming worthlessness of life. It plunges one into a darkness where everything is black, but it is the darkness of the chrysalis, a place of disintegration that will provide the substance of new life. The very basis of existence as we have known it begins to crumble. The values and ideals of youth no longer speak, and we are deeply disturbed, or even horrified, at what becomes apparent. 'I seemed to be in a snake pit with all my fears, powerlessness, confusion and despair writhing in a sort of macabre dance within me,' one member of a workshop wrote. 'I felt I had lost all meaning in life and yet, strangely enough, in spite of all this there was a spark of hope.' Some do not see this 'spark of hope'. They become so trapped in the mire of the transition that the rest of their lives is spent battling with its conflicting aspects.

All that has been spoken of in dealing with crises applies to this transition, but for each one it shows a different face. Listlessness, apathy, a loss of interest or involvement in work may be all that some experience. While others find the very foundations of life falling away. Feelings of anger, regret, self-doubt and resentment may suffocate them. Or again, they may be paralysed by a sense of unease, withdrawal or of being caught in some relentless trap.

Entry into the afternoon of life gives rise to a re-appraisal of all that has gone before with a questioning of every aspect of the past. Career and professional life are usually the first areas to come under scrutiny for men. A growing frustration, a sense of being used or of failing ability can lead to a deepening dissatisfaction with the current occupation. If, as is so often the case, self-worth has been tied to production, this stress, and the added one of time running out, may give rise to overactivity. The attempt to compensate for the apparent lack of achievement rarely succeeds. If it continues, burnout will inevitably result. A similar picture leading to burnout is often seen in women whether in the workforce or in the home, but this tends to occur later in the crisis and not to initiate it.

Just as women found their identity through relating intimately with another, it is frequently in the area of relationships that they first feel the discontent and self-delusion that marks the entry into mid-life. The deepening of their power of intimacy, especially self-intimacy, is preceded by a change in self-image, and for a period this gives rise to disruption in their ability to relate. Feelings of loneliness, of being out of touch with others, of isolation and doubt as to their own loveableness weigh heavily on many. The emotional instability of this time of life also brings about a swing in both men and women between infatuation, similar to that of adolescence, and alienation: between a falling in love and a falling out of love.

For many, self-exploration leads to serious questioning of vocation or career. Doubt as to the wisdom of an original choice is emphasised by the negatives which are becoming apparent. This re-assessment is a healthy indicator that the level of commitment is undergoing necessary change. It may require a period of standing back, a respite or moratorium, before it is possible to see clearly where we are being called.

The re-evaluation at this time of life not infrequently results in a change of occupation and a re-expression of one's earlier desires. Or it may serve to reassure that the initial choice remains the most suitable one. Gerald O'Collins speaks of these second journeys taking the form of either an Aeneid or an Odyssey.[6] Do we, with Aeneas or perhaps with Abraham, find our journey takes us to new and unexplored terrain? Or are we led with Ulysses, or with Moses, to the land which was always truly ours?

The mid-point of life's journey is above all a moment when the whole context of faith or a philosophy of life is re-examined. What has been received from parents, teachers, friends must now become our own, a belief to which we can pledge an allegiance as mature adults.

The transition from a given religious faith to a committed one is part of the struggle in the mid-life crisis. It is accompanied by confusion, doubt, and often aridity, as we strive to determine what to let go and what to retain. For the most part God seems strangely absent in this conflict, silent, aloof and unheeding of our predicament. The discrepancy between what we had hoped to be at this stage of life and what we have become often haunts us. Sinfulness becomes an acknowledged part of this reality. The recognition of human weakness can bring with it an oppressive burden of guilt and it requires courage to face and to accept such frailty. For some this struggle proves to be the darkest point of the mid-life transition. As they wrestle to leave behind their idols of perfection and embrace fully the human condition which is theirs, they are moving from the discipleship of youth to the mature stewardship of the Kingdom. This is the moment of conversion.

For those who do not adhere to a religious faith, a similar struggle can be experienced as they re-examine the philosophy which up until now has directed their lives. Doubt as to the validity of previous attitudes may overwhelm them as they, too, wrestle to reach a more appropriate outlook on life.

The mid-life crisis is indeed the most vital of all the transitions. It ushers in a new and fuller way of life discovered in the exploration of the world we hold within. The depth of confusion and the degree of pain experienced are no more than indicators of the measure of hope for the afternoon of life. If we can allow ourselves to register and feel these emotions, and not repress or deny them, they herald a future full of promise.

♦ ♦ ♦

Chapter • 4

MID-LIFE DEVELOPMENTAL TASKS

The passage through the mid-life transition can be one of confusion, of being out of touch with oneself, even of a painful bordering on despair. Finally, however, there lies ahead a quieter and less tumultuous stage which Levinson calls 'Entering Middle Adulthood'. The call to individuation continues, and the tasks already commenced during the time of crisis still go on. The psychologists mentioned earlier describe in detail what is central to this period.

For Jung, the afternoon of life is now beginning and noon is left behind. He asserts that 'we cannot live the afternoon of life according to the programme of life's morning; what was great in the morning will be little in the evening; what in the morning was true, in the evening will have become a lie'.[1] There is a gradual change of attitude, with new perceptions and deeper levels of understanding. This is the moment that we begin to take on the full responsibility for our own lives. To see that, perhaps despite a difficult home background with abusive or unloving parents, we are ultimately responsible for what we become. As one mid-lifer, who for a long time had found refuge in blaming the conditions of her early life for the way she was acting, said: 'I can now see my mother could not have been different. She herself was an abused child and was not even able to get the help that I have. It is for me to make my own life what I want it to be.' For many, this can be the moment of forgiveness of parents and a reconciliation which is life-giving to both.

The second phase of the process of individuation, bringing into balance the opposite sides of the personality, is slowly taking place with the advent of the forties. Now the psyche intuitively aspires to an equilibrium. But this cannot happen fully without a sustained involvement in our inner world, a getting to know ourselves at depth. The Maori people of New Zealand have a symbol, often carved on the bows of their canoes, the koru: 'haere mai' — being the 'come inward', make the journey within, and the 'haere atu', 'go forth', carry with you what you have received. This is a message which men and women at mid-life would do well to heed.

The journey inward is not a self-centred movement but seeks rather to develop the Self in relation to the community. It requires time and the necessary space to allow the developing sense of interiority to lead us beyond the self-knowledge already possessed. The middle years are so often frenetically busy years as new responsibilities in work or family present themselves. For some the sort of space needed is a luxury which they find beyond their reach. It may be only later in life that they are able to undertake this inner journey.

The movement within to discover who one really is brings the person face to face, not only with the good, but also with the dark aspect, the unwanted or undeveloped part of the personality. Jung gives the name, the shadow, to this archetypal side. It is the reverse of all that one has chosen to be in the first part of life. It consists of the many aspects of the personality rejected or denied as one strives to develop a persona agreeable to others, or to give expression to preferred values and ideals. Unwanted and forgotten, these negative aspects live on in the unconscious, becoming part of the personal shadow. But the shadow is not all dark; it has a brighter side. It consists also of the positive qualities and aptitudes which have never been developed, for a variety of reasons, and now await recognition and acceptance.

The growing awareness of this part of the personality can be an overwhelming and painful experience as over the years we meet more and more of the qualities which earlier we had chosen to ignore. But, as Jung stresses, 'new meaning for life is so often found in the inferior and undeveloped side of the personality'.[2] Within the shadow can be concealed great riches, pure gold. Many abilities and skills which have lain dormant, can emerge and if cultivated, will enrich the whole of life, while the more negative traits, when recognised, can be directed into an acceptable expression. Once owned and named these less desired elements of the personality are far more readily controlled. 'Many, far too many, aspects of life which should have been experienced lie in the lumber-room among dusty memories. Sometimes, even, they are glowing coals under grey ashes.'[3] A great deal of energy is also tied up in the shadow and will be liberated for use in other areas when this aspect of ourselves can be acknowledged.

How does this hidden side reveal itself? It can do so in several ways. It may appear in dreams, or fantasies, be met in projections or heard through an inner voice.

At this stage of life, dream figures of the same sex as the dreamer are frequently messengers from the unconscious, revealing something of the shadow and the need to recognise and accept it. The shadow appears most often as a person who is in some way inferior, and whom we despise, dread or even fear. Janet related a dream in which she was walking contentedly through a peaceful and beautiful forest when suddenly she came upon a little log cabin in a clearing. She went in and felt immediately at home. This was her place, strong and safe. As she gazed through the window she saw a wild and dishevelled old hag approaching the door. Immediately she closed it, barring it with a large bolt attached to the wood with screws. As the woman started beating on the door to be let in, she saw to her horror that the screws attaching the bolt were gradually loosening. She was terrified. As the bolt gave way a woman in tattered, dirty clothing stood before her. The woman simply laughed and disappeared and Janet felt all her dread drain rapidly away. In discussing this dream, Janet, a perfectionist in every way including dress, became aware that this was her shadow wanting to be acknowledged. The wild, uncontrolled, untidy part of her personality had never been allowed to surface as she held herself a prisoner in the bonds of her own perfectionism. With the recognition of this hidden side, she moved into a freedom which 'no longer cared so much about appearances'. The laughter of the woman in the dream is not unusual, as humour is closely associated with the shadow. 'Wherever there is humour the shadow is involved,'[4] John Sanford informs us.

An even more common revelation of the shadow is through projection. There is in all of us a tendency to project onto others, to see in them those traits, desirable or undesirable, which we fail to recognise in ourselves. Projection is the defence mechanism used to protect oneself against the ownership of such qualities. We attempt, as W.A. Miller says, 'to throw them away'.[5] But they cannot be disposed of as easily as that. Instead they are seen mirrored in someone else of the same sex who provides sufficient reason for the projection. Unwanted traits are thrown onto the hook that that person provides by showing something of the same weaknesses, or sometimes strengths. Projection is recognised when we find ourselves over-reacting, becoming unduly upset or, perhaps, fascinated by this aspect of our shadow in another. 'The projection ceases,' according to Jung, 'the moment it becomes conscious, that is to say, when it is seen as belonging to the subject.'[6] Once this has been accepted it can be mastered. For example, instead of being intensely irritated by what appears to be manipulation by another, we are obliged to recognise the ways in which we are unwittingly manipulative. Only then is it possible to correct this defect. Morton Kelsey claims that whenever we make a projection conscious and are willing to take responsibility for it, it becomes the highest form of prayer.

What is concealed from us is often blatantly obvious to those who know us. Valuable information about the hidden self can come from those closest to us, especially in moments when their guard is down or they speak to us in anger. It is good to take time to look at what has been said and to search for the truth that may be there, though it will rarely prove easy to accept and own it.

Slips of the tongue, when what is said is different from what was intended, or conversations with an inner voice, can also reveal aspects of the shadow.

These are ways in which perhaps a hidden resentment, hostility or envy is revealed. One married man was left with much to ponder when, while discussing mid-life, 'wild life' slipped out instead.

Once recognised, these denied aspects of the personality can find expression in ways that are not overly disruptive. Unrecognised and unowned, they tend to bubble up and erupt in a way that can be destructive both to the person concerned and to others. Accepted for what they are, they can add an enriching dimension to relationships. Just as a landscape without shadow is a flat and uninspiring picture, so, too, is someone without human flaws a tasteless and insipid companion. The person who accepts his or her shadow is a person of substance. To deny the shadow is to deny reality, to become unreal, a fake.

Jung stresses the need, at this time of life, and indeed through the whole of life to be open to our shadow side, not to fear it. We are all human and must have human weaknesses, and, for various reasons, part of our personality will have been left undeveloped. It is for us now to acknowledge this, to befriend the shadow, accepting it as an essential part of our total personality.

These middle years are also a time of expansion of the conscious psyche, a time when much that has been previously unconscious begins to surface into consciousness. Not only do many memories come back to haunt, or perhaps to fascinate us, but archetypes, only vaguely recognised in earlier life, begin to manifest themselves more clearly. Among these are the contrasexual aspects of the person to which Jung gives the names animus and anima. 'Every man carries within him the eternal image of woman, not the image of this or that woman but a definite feminine image ... I have called this image the anima

... The same is true of the woman: she too has her inborn image of the man, the animus.'[7] These archetypes spring originally from the collective unconscious and are coloured by the individual's experience of the opposite sex: mother or father, brother or sister, or people met during the earlier years of life. One of the tasks confronted on the journey towards wholeness is the integration into the conscious personality of these sexually opposite aspects, which have not previously been fully recognised for a combination of biological and cultural reasons.

Biologically there would seem to be a difference in the natural personality traits of men and women, though this has proved difficult to confirm scientifically. However, it is obvious that society has come to expect certain characteristics of women or of men. These are not inherent in their primary sexuality, maleness or femaleness, but are rather culturally determined and are referred to as masculine or feminine traits. Society encourages children to develop, from the first, in ways it considers as 'appropriate' to their sex. Many qualities, such as aggressiveness and toughness are usually tolerated or even encouraged in little boys, whereas the gentler qualities are fostered in the girl. The child soon learns the sometimes unspoken message that there is a fitting way to behave and urges to the contrary should be suppressed. So it is that instead of developing the whole scope of possibilities in the first half of life, we tend to favour either the culturally masculine or feminine attributes.

The characteristics generally spoken of as masculine are those governed by the logos or rational principle, for example focused consciousness, objectivity, logicality and analytic thinking. The ability to manipulate things, to break them into parts for analysis and to compartmentalise life all belong to the masculine principle. This tends to be more expressive and assertive. Those traits referred to as feminine are directed rather by eros, the principle of relatedness and union, and are more receptive. These include a diffuse awareness facilitating the ability to see connections, intuition, empathy and gentleness. The feminine relates readily to persons and tends to perceive things as wholes. The masculine elements are embodied for the woman in the animus; the feminine for the man in the anima. As John Welch explains them: 'The anima is that which sees relationships, makes whole, values and reaches out. The animus refers to the ability to discriminate, focus, differentiate and define.'[8] As women become more readily accepted in various fields of activity, many of the traits belonging to the animus are integrated in the earlier part of life, and some men also begin to integrate the more feminine aspects in early adulthood.

On the whole, however, it is with the advent of the middle years that the qualities embodied in the animus or anima become more apparent. Strangely, it would seem that the negative qualities of this archetype are usually the first to make their presence felt. The man may find himself becoming more irritable, temperamental or touchy, as the anima stirs into consciousness. Reluctant to accept these moods, he will often try to suppress them again. He will then tend, quite unconsciously, to project these undesirable qualities onto the first appropriate woman he encounters. This is often his wife. Only later do the more attractive qualities of the anima surface. Again, if he does not accept this side of his personality, a second projection may occur. This time it will not be on the woman already carrying his first projection but probably on someone outside his family, perhaps his secretary or assistant. She will then become the charming and alluring presence in his life.

The emergence of this archetype in the man is frequently associated with an upsurge of sexual fantasies and erotic desires. A fascination with erotica may herald the movement to consciousness of the anima, that eros-governed aspect of his nature. This can serve as a message to the mid-life man that the time has come to accept and integrate that part of his whole personality which, in earlier years, he has been forced to put aside. The challenge now is to be receptive to the gifts which are being offered to him, of care and relatedness to his inner world, of gentleness and openness to his affectivity.

For the woman, the animus presents not so much the image of one man but of 'man' in general and often appears in dreams as a group of men. Its influence at first is frequently a negative one. Whereas the anima is, in Sanford's words, 'the master of moods in a man', the animus is the 'master of opinions in a woman'.[9] Those rather harsh and opinionated views which invade a woman's thoughts and are so often voiced in authoritative statements, no matter how irrelevant or incorrect, spring from her animus. Their origin is not in her own thinking or feeling, but rather in what has come to her from various authority figures throughout life. Jung speaks of the animus as the source of 'an inexhaustible supply of illogical arguments and false explanations'.[10] The positive aspect of the animus is seen in the way it enables the woman to recognise more clearly the gifts she already holds within and to be more assertive in their expression. As Irene De Castillejo explains: 'The woman needs the animus' torch (focusing power) to light up for her the things she innately knows, so that she can know that she knows them.'[11]

The meeting with the animus and the anima is, in

the words of Jung, 'the masterpiece of individuation'.[12] This does not mean that the animus or anima should be allowed to dominate the personality. Rather to avoid this, the man or woman must first identify the revelations of these archetypes which come to him or her through projections, dreams, fantasies or from inner voices. Once recognised and owned the important work of integration begins.

For the man it becomes important to differentiate between the moods which may overwhelm him and his own true feelings. The former are from the anima, the latter from his affective life. If his feelings are acknowledged and given expression in a human relationship he will not be dominated by his moods, but led by his anima into a closer relatedness with others. The woman too must keep aware of her own values and judgements and not allow the negative animus to foist false or critical ideas upon her. The positive animus will then 'light up' for her her own true values and worth and lead her to a possession of them, possibly for the first time in her life.

From the above it can be seen that if these archetypal figures are ignored or neglected they can wreak havoc in our lives. Acknowledged and welcomed they are guides leading us deeply into our inner world. The animus and anima are the link between the conscious and the unconscious. They help us to feel and relate more fully or to think and reflect more clearly, thus directing us on the journey of individuation.

Central to this journey is the meeting with the Self, the archetype of wholeness and the final revealer of our true and full personality. We have seen that individuation at this stage of life requires the integration or accepting and owning of both sides of the personality: the unconscious as well as the conscious, the dark side as well as the light, the masculine together with the feminine, and all the opposites which are gradually rising to consciousness. It is the Self that strives to bring balance and harmony between these different elements. But this will only be achieved when the ego, centre of the conscious personality, can let go of the values it has held to so strongly for the first half of life. The struggle can be bitter and must be faced at many levels before finally the ego recognises its rightful place in the service of the Self. Thus the Self assumes its central role. One client related a dream in which she found herself struggling to give birth in a long and difficult labour. After what she described as hours of painful stress, she became aware of a tiny new-born baby lying by her side. She felt a powerful love fill her whole being. As she bent to pick up and nurse the child 'it melted into her heart'. This woman had been experiencing a tremendous struggle to accept the person she was beginning to recognise within. She came to realise, through this dream, that the new Self, as yet so fragile, must be the centre which she loved and nurtured.

The same theme is taken up by Levinson when he discusses the need to bring about a new balance between the many opposite aspects of our personalities. He describes the main work of mid-life as a rebalancing of four major polarities: the Young/Old, Destruction/Creation, Masculine/Feminine and Attachment/Separateness.

Of these four he sees the Young/Old as central. We are, at every stage of life, both young and old. The new-born baby may be an hour or even a day old; the old man still holds within him many of the qualities of youth. These qualities speak to all of us of adventure, energy, enthusiasm, idealism and openness to future possibilities, while those of old age suggest rather completion, stability, fruition and the wisdom gained from experience. The passage into the afternoon of life brings with it the need to learn appropriate ways of retaining youth while at the same time accepting the fact of ageing and acting accordingly. There are those who refuse to recognise this and resist letting go of the manifestations of youth that they have known. Who has not met the mid-life 'Peter Pan' or the one who hopes to 'jog' his years into oblivion? The challenge, then, is to face the inevitability of ageing while allowing it to be energised by the youth which remains within. 'I am uneasy at heart,' Tagore confesses, 'when I have to leave my accustomed shelter, I forget there abides the old in the new, and that there also thou abidest.'[13] We must be willing to recognise the limits imposed by our years, while at the same time welcoming the growing inner power and authority which is ours. From the middle of life onwards, Jung tells us, only those who are ready to die with life will remain vitally alive; only those who are willing to accept the necessary losses in life will live life to its fullest.

The diminishments felt at mid-life often bring one face to face with the realisation of mortality and with it a fear of approaching death. Elliott Jaques, an English psychologist, stresses that this fear may be the focal point of mid-life for many. The loss in death, perhaps of parents or close friends, confronts us with the realisation of our own finiteness. The struggle to come to terms with this can grow intense. It is difficult to face the possibility of the end of life when youth's desire for immortality is still so strongly with us. It is the wish for immortality which inspires the man or woman at this time of life to work to leave behind something of value, a legacy which will enrich the lives of the following generation.

Mid-life grieving for the many losses experienced is

a common phenomenon. The loss of youth, or reproductive ability, perhaps of figure, and of children from the home, are all traumatic events in the lives of most. We readily appreciate the pain and loneliness so often felt by a mother in the home who sees her children leave one by one until she is left with a large and empty house. The loss experienced by the working mother or father is sometimes overlooked. Having spent long hours during the children's early years earning the means to ensure schooling and recreation, they have looked forward to a time when this pressure will be eased. When at last there is space to enjoy the companionship of the family, it can come as a bitter blow that adolescent sons and daughters are now ready to leave home and find their independence.

As in the case of all loss, we need to allow time for the process of grieving. Then from it a new found peace will grow.

There is also a new awareness of time and a shift in its perception. Whereas previously time was of little consequence and tended to stretch out almost endlessly ahead, it now becomes a precious commodity which is limited and seems to be rapidly running out. Time-left becomes more important than time-since-birth and a sense of urgency is often felt. As one woman put it: 'I feel pressured in a way I never did before. There is so much still to do and time simply vanishes.'

The man and woman in the mid years become more and more aware of the multiple destructive forces both within themselves and in the world around them. There is often a feeling of powerlessness to alleviate this. But at the same time they are conscious of creative powers stirring within and a growing sense of inner strength. According to Levinson: 'Both sides of the Destruction/Creation polarity are intensified at mid-life. The acute sense of his own ultimate destruction intensifies a man's wish for creation. His growing wish to be creative is accompanied by a greater awareness of the destructive forces in nature, in human life generally, and in himself.'[14] In a world of atomic power, of the natural disasters of flood and famine, of conflict and discord in the family, both men and women are challenged to conceive new and creative responses to the destructive forces which surround us on every side.

How many men and women devote much of their energy to social causes for the betterment of the world that is theirs. Perhaps we are, for the first time, beginning to assume responsibility for the planet on which we live. 'You become responsible, forever, for what you have tamed,'[15] the fox once told the Little Prince. The peace movements and the many ecological societies are but a few examples of the efforts being made to reverse the devastation of the land. They are evidence of a new awakening to this obligation to preserve, enhance and beautify our world.

Recognition dawns, too, that each one has been touched personally by similar destructive forces. Not only do we become aware of the harm we have done to others, but also see more clearly how they may have damaged us, in childhood, or the earlier years of work or marriage. Mid-life is a time to face the hurts and injustices of the first half of life and to come to terms with the feelings of anger, resentment or guilt which are hidden deep within. As attitudes change, we will discover new ways of expressing these emotions without injury to others.

Healing of memories plays an important part during these years and will be referred to again in a later chapter. Enough to say here that unless we can open ourselves to these feelings and not continue to deny them, the possibility of becoming generative, creative and loving will be severely restricted.

Many find their healing comes through a growing urge to be creative. Their pain and confusion is often spilled out in poetry or painting. Some of the world's most renowned artists produced their greatest masterpieces as they struggled to give expression to both the destruction and creation polarities. Milton's 'Paradise Lost' found its source in the distress of losing his sight at the age of forty-two. T.S. Eliot in describing his struggle 'in the middle way ... trying to learn to use words' wrote

And each new venture
Is a new beginning, a raid on the inarticulate
With shabby equipment always deteriorating
In the general mess of imprecision of feeling,
Undisciplined squads of emotion.[16]

The artist, Gaugin, escaped from the drudgery and boredom of his life as a Paris broker at forty-five. He found new vitality and spirit through his paintings of the people of Tahiti. Closer to home, many mid-life men and women are discovering exciting, untapped talent in the music, art and literary centres of adult education.

Not all have such artistic abilities, but at least they can search for fresh and creative ways of approaching a family problem or dealing with an impasse at the office or factory bench. New ideas and the urge to bring a better quality of life to others have led many to join welfare organisations or establish care and concern groups at this stage of life.

In dealing with the Masculine/Feminine polarity Levinson discusses the necessity for men to allow the feminine to play a 'larger and freer part' in their lives; to develop their sensitivity and to be more in touch with their capacity to relate. In the case of women it is the moment to recognise and give expression to a growing inner strength; to be more assertive and confident in taking charge of their lives. We have already seen, while looking at the encounter with the animus and anima, much of what this adaptation entails, and how difficult it can prove for many.

Levinson speaks finally of the necessity to rework the Attachment/Separateness polarity. He underlines here the need to 'reduce a heavy involvement in the external world'[17] in order to give space to enter more deeply within in the discovery of the true Self. For the person who has not developed a capacity for separateness, space to be alone with oneself, the prospect can be a daunting one. A rebalancing of the desire for intimacy and involvement with that for solitude or aloneness must again take place. Not only has our involvement with others been one of career or friendship, but there has also been a strong dependency on the standards, views and judgements imposed by parents, teachers and the outside world in general. As we uncover inner strengths and resources, we become less bound by the expectations of others, the 'shoulds' and 'oughts' of childhood and the approval of the outside world. We reach a new freedom and a security in our own values and opinions. Self-doubt and the need for constant affirmation from others gives way to a sense of worth, fitting us to achieve a better balance between personal needs and those of the society in which we live.

We experience other personality changes at this time as the result of a strengthening of the psychological functions which up until now have remained less well developed. Jung speaks of the powers of thinking, feeling, intuiting and sensing. He maintains that from early life one particular process has been preferred as the way in which we spontaneously respond to the world. Because of some basic orientation within, we trust and develop one way of acting more strongly than the others. In the second half of life, the less developed functions start to seek attention. Imperceptibly they are integrated and used more readily, without, however, a change in our basic orientation. Maturity will depend on our ability to integrate these opposites into our way of contacting reality.

Jung sees that personalities differ, too, according to their fundamental attitudes of either extraversion or introversion. Some find themselves energised and enthused by the world around them; others find their source of energy within. The former are the extraverts of the world; the latter, the introverts. It is important to understand that introverts at any stage of life can be quite out-going people, even though some tend to be withdrawn. Extraverts can also be reflective but are drawn to invest energy in their environment and surroundings. The introvert is said to reflect both before and after action; the extravert acts more spontaneously, or even impulsively, and reflects afterwards. These basic attitudes tend to reach a better balance in the middle years.

We find a powerful means of assisting in the integration of these previously hidden and undeveloped parts of the personality in the ability to play. Play facilitates integration and individuation, for in it 'we let go of the consciousness that directs our energies and experience whole other areas of our being'.[18] Its importance is often overlooked in this second part of life. In the late twenties and thirties the pressures to succeed, to make a niche in the world, frequently leave little space for leisure or relaxation. Gradually, we can fail to find a place in our lives for play. And we become the poorer for this. There is no time to delight in nature or to laugh at one's own or others' foibles. The book of Proverbs tells that Wisdom, the joyful companion of God, 'is ever at play in his presence, at play everywhere in his world' (Proverbs, 8:30-31). Those who can play this way in his presence, will be much more open to receive the gift of wisdom. For play puts us in touch with the wellspring of laughter and fun and fosters a gentle wit which will lead ultimately into the wisdom of the aged. There is a strong link, too, between creativity and play. The relaxed mind is freed to listen to the spontaneous promptings of imagination. It can then give expression to these inspirations in ways that are novel and inventive.

The quality of play at this time of life is often different from that of the younger person. It becomes less success-oriented and competitive, more relaxing and enjoyable; it presupposes a level of trust and a capacity for relating. 'In play,' George Vaillant points out, 'we must trust enough and love enough to risk losing without despair, to bear winning without guilt and to laugh at error without mockery.'[19] In play, we meet once more the spontaneous, fun-loving child who lives on in the depths of each of us and will lead us to a new-found freedom and joy.

♦ ♦ ♦

Chapter • 5

THE GENERATIVE PERSON

The culmination of the mid-life tasks, according to Erikson, is the development of generativity. This is the quality which inspires a person who is in touch with his or her identity and is able to relate intimately with another, to be more concerned now with enriching the lives of others. It is the positive outcome of the struggle against becoming ensnared in narcissistic preoccupations as we are drawn into our inner world.

The 'heightened importance of introspection and increased interiority of the person at mid-life'[1] is appropriate and necessary for the entry into the afternoon of life. It will persist as afternoon fades into evening. As it deepens, it effects a lessening in self-centredness and a broadening of focus to embrace others. The psychological power facilitating this transcendence of self is what Erikson has named the 'vital strength' of care which is 'the widening concern for what has been generated by love, necessity or accident'.[2] It is a non-possessive love and solicitude which encourages the other to come to a full possession of his or her own identity and latent possibilities.

Our generative care is directed strongly to the younger generation to ensure for them a quality of life which will help them reach their full potential. But this same care is frequently also addressed to the preceding generation. A new quality of concern is found in the solicitude shown to the requirements of ageing or ailing parents, friends and those in need. The middle-aged son or daughter so often assumes the role of concerned carer for a failing father or mother.

Failure to meet the demands of this particular crisis of generativity results in an inability to see beyond one's own requirements, to become stagnant or self-absorbed. Either narcissistic or depressed individuals most frequently evade the effort needed for satisfactory integration during this turning point of life. Should this be the case, the former tend to become more and more occupied with acquiring material possessions and less and less willing to share them with others. Their concern with acquaintances can be measured by what they hope to obtain from them. Such individuals may undergo a complete change in perspective if serious illness or some misfortune forces them to recognise their dependence on others. This 'conversion' can lead to a mellowing in old age and a reversal of the state of stagnation. As the result of hospitalisation after a heart attack, one cantankerous elderly man was transformed by what he spoke of as 'the real thoughtfulness' of the nursing staff.

The depressed, however, who slip into self-absorption, do not usually undergo this change. Such individuals see themselves as having nothing worthwhile to offer others. Their pessimism and poor self-image only increase as the years go by until inevitably they find themselves in the despair of old age, the dystonic disposition of life's final crisis. It is sad to see the relatively common picture of an old person immersed in a sense of worthlessness and self-pity.

To become absorbed in oneself in this way can lead to 'an obsessive need for pseudo-intimacy . . . often with a pervading sense of stagnation and personal impoverishment.'[3] There is no mature or genuine mutuality in the give and take of a relationship in one who fails to negotiate this crisis, for the power of self-giving is lost.

Generative adulthood, however, is ready to take on the responsibilities of nurturing, maintaining and furthering life, whether it be of children, ideas, projects or whatever is the product of creativity. This is what we understand by being willing to assume a stewardship of life, a readiness to support, to guide and to lead what has been produced to its own eventual maturity and independence.

It is only the person who has satisfactorily integrated and adequately re-worked each of Erikson's epigenetic stages who will reach the fullness of generative adulthood.

In this beginning of life's afternoon there is a change in orientation, and the ego spoken of by Jung gives way to the control of the emergent Self. The integration completed in the earlier part of life must be worked through once more, this time in relationship to our inner world rather than to the world around us. This re-integration is vital to the development of generativity.

The basic trust in the conscious aspects of life, first developed in infancy, must extend to a confidence in the second personality emerging from the depths of our unconscious psyche, the new person we are becoming. This trust will be apparent, too, in a strong faith in the meaningfulness of life, expressed for some in a religious context, for others, perhaps, in a philosophical one.[4]

The autonomy of early childhood changes into a sense of self-assurance as renewed doubt at mid-life leads us to relinquish many previously held perceptions. No longer are we so threatened by a fear of failure. We can stand firm in support of the opinions and principles important to us without being unduly rigid or opinionated. Justice both to oneself and others will become central to the judgments and involvements undertaken. This sense of independence and autonomy leads many at this stage of life to commit themselves to causes which give expression to their deep convictions. It is not unusual to find someone, who would previously never have dared speak in public, addressing large gatherings on valued convictions without self-consciousness or fear.

The initiative and purpose which emerged in the play age must be reworked as the shadow within is met and integrated. As the ideals and goals of earlier life are renegotiated, the mature adult acquires a fresh vision. There is a drive to bring new projects into being and to carry through to fulfilment what has been started. The desire to leave a legacy for the next generation grows strong. The former 'harsh conscience of childhood'[5] also gives way to a mature appreciation of right values and choices.

A sense of competence and capability will promote a healthy self-esteem as we struggle again with the sense of emptiness and uselessness which eroded our self-image during the crisis of mid-life. It was only constant reassurances that her own sense of uselessness might be of help to others that enabled Barbara, widowed at forty-eight, to become a quietly competent and empathic teacher of the disabled. This in turn led to the reinforcement of her own self-confidence and finally to a real conviction of her worth.

The generative adult will have acquired a firm sense of identity as he or she comes to terms with the new emerging personality of the second half of life. This results in the ability 'to sustain loyalties freely pledged in spite of the inevitable contradictions of value systems'.[6] It will allow for a freedom in assuming a variety of roles and relationships without confusion or dissipation of the Self. It is this 'self-possession' which allows and motivates many leaders in our society to be involved in a multitude of business, civic and charitable enterprises without undue stress or exhaustion.

And, finally, as the intimacy crisis is re-worked in mid-life it gives rise to a capacity to relate at new depths not only to others but to oneself as well. Our closeness to others is always in direct proportion to our ability to know and relate with appreciation to ourselves, to be at ease and comfortable with our feelings and insights. This implies a readiness for sexual intimacy in a continued commitment of love without threat to the newly found Self. It also implies a true mutuality between mature friends with no loss of personal boundaries. The experience of deepening intimacy with another has a profound impact on our ability to relate closely and freely with God. The successful re-facing of this crisis also involves, as Fowler tells us, 'a readiness to engage in conflict without withdrawal or the need to destroy the opponent, and sustains one in situations of shared inspiration and creation'.[7]

The appropriate re-working of all these earlier stages is vital to the development at mid-life of a strong sense of responsibility for the nurture and welfare of what has been produced in life's morning. Generativity is the fruit of the re-integration of all six strengths gained in the early stages of development combined with successfully resisting the mire of self-absorption. For women, who may have become generative at a much earlier stage, there still remains the task of resolving this crisis in a way expressive of their maturity in the second half of life.

The generative adult will find countless ways to express the wealth of concern burgeoning within. Middle-aged parents are often faced with the need to 'let go' of teenage children as they seek to develop their own potential outside the home-circle. True care will allow the young to risk and grow through their mistakes without parents being overprotective or possessive.

We find a genuine expression of love in the willingness to receive from others as well as to give. To accept help, kindness or concern from another means to surrender the dominant position, which rests always with the giver, and to allow the other to take that position towards us.

We may express solicitude towards others through some outreach into community services or into the network of charitable organisations we find in our society. Some of us may seek to leave a legacy to the next generation through an institution or project of enduring relevance, others to assume an advisory role or a directorship of an already established organisation. 'Generativity is itself a driving power in human organisation,'[8] Erikson assures us.

Many of the older generation adopt a relationship of mentor, supporting and guiding a younger person in a chosen career or vocation; sharing the fruit of their own experience to enrich another. This must be done with care and without attempting to manipulate in any way. The mentor should always be prepared to relinquish the relationship when the younger person is ready to move to independence. This is usually somewhere within the first decade of the association. Failure to do so can lead to much anguish and hurt for the older person who may well feel rejected or unwanted when help is no longer sought. In fact, such a person has simply completed the task he or she set out to do, and must now leave the next generation to the independence which was, after all, the real goal of this mentorship. The appropriate relationship then becomes one of mutuality, but the shift to this is usually not without its traumas and misunderstandings.

Women, in particular, experience the maturing of generativity as a growing sense of inner power and a readiness to be assertive in the service of their own well-being, as well as that of others. Lives that have been spent till now in caring for family, pupils, patients or clients may well make claims for the recognition and respect of personal needs at this moment. Talents may cry out for development, skills call for some expression beyond the home, office or classroom. A new independence and freedom is discovered, as many women, and some men, find their way at this stage of life into universities, colleges and schools of art, or become involved in planning in local or higher government. The desire is there, in both women and men, to give of their own accumulated experience for the betterment of a world which will continue after they have gone. As one person expressed it: 'I am concerned to teach others as much as I can of what I myself have learnt.'[9]

The truly generative have learnt, as Peck points out, to value wisdom over physical prowess, 'putting the use of their heads above the use of their hands as their standard for self-evaluation and as their chief source of solving life's problems'.[10] They have come to appreciate individual characteristics as more important in relationships than sexual prowess and thereby have often deepened such relationships. They have attained an emotional flexibility, enabling them to 'shift emotional investments from one person to another and from one activity to another'.[11] This does not imply an emotional instability but rather an ability to re-adjust emotionally at this stage of life when they can expect the loss of children, often the death of friends and sometimes spouse or partner. This is also the time that most people will have acquired the widest circle and the broadest age-range of friends and business acquaintances that they will ever encounter.

Finally, the generative person is one who has kept a mental flexibility, who remains open to new ideas, can listen to and learn from others and has not become set in past ways, inflexible or rigid in thought or opinion.

The years of mid-life are the ideal time for community or church leadership.[12] The man or woman who has matured successfully through the middle years has acquired a sense of responsibility combined with the willingness to delegate, to hand over to others where appropriate, to recognise limits and yet to have the self-confidence to hold firmly to tested ideals and values. They can blend competence with concern, assertiveness with gentleness and empathy.

The person at mid-life is well suited to assume the mantle of leadership. Our streets and church pews are filled with those both willing and able to offer their services in this way for the good of their society. They can bring to their leadership a spirit of hope, a competence derived from many years of experience, a willingness to support the weak and a compassion born of their own sufferings.

Generativity and the care that accompanies it opens

us to a new involvement in living, a fresh enjoyment of the simple things around us, a love of all that is beautiful and a renewed awe at the wonders of nature. It gives rise to an inner peace as we learn to accept with realism the limits of life and to face the years of ageing that lie before us.

Generativity preludes the advent of wisdom. It is out of the pain and trauma of accepting our own limitedness that springs the capacity to be a bearer of life and hope to others.

A story was told in ancient China of a war-lord who from earliest childhood was trained to be ruler. He lived in great luxury with servants to answer his every need, and a loyal army to quell his enemies and to keep order in his realm. He was powerful and knew himself to be a just, if harsh, man. When he rode out amongst them, his people would, in respect, turn their faces to the wall so that he never saw the ravages of disease, hunger and starvation amongst those who could no longer work in his fields. In his own life he knew nothing of such things.

Then a neighbouring enemy who coveted his rich rice paddies and cultivated fields gathered a vast army and took possession of the kingdom. The conquered war-lord was cast into prison with the lowest dregs of humankind. Bound and locked in a dingy cell, he saw himself again astride his war horse riding freely through the length of his domain. He thought of what others had told him of the sick of his kingdom, unable to stir from their pallets in the shabby dwellings by his cultivated fields; and he knew the suffering of imprisonment. When his gaolers brought him his daily portion of mouldy rice and stale tea, he remembered his feasting and then he recalled his labourers' meagre rations and he began to understand their hunger. His mat on the bare floor was hard but he thought then of the wretched pallets of his poorest subjects.

Years later as a mark of largesse, a new ruler in his conqueror's kingdom ordered all prisoners released. The war-lord, broken and humbled by his years of imprisonment, returned unknown to his own country and settled in a vacant hovel for now he had no claim to his palace or riches. A sympathetic neighbour let him sow a little rice in a small, no longer fertile patch. Yet he managed to raise enough to satisfy his meagre needs, and even had a little over. This he gave to the family of a sick man because he remembered what it was to be starving.

In time, the old war-lord-turned-beggar persuaded others of the labourers to help those who could no longer provide for their children and the sick who could not leave their pallets. Joy spread in this area of the slums as people started to care for each other, to share with those who did not have enough. And the old man moved among his people grieving for their sorrow, feeling the pain of their hunger, and the isolation of their loneliness. As war-lord he had ruled with justice, but there was no joy in his kingdom. Now through his brokenness and poverty he had become a source of hope and life, a true leader of his people.

♦ ♦ ♦

Chapter • 6

STRESS AND BURNOUT

Today's world is filled with pressures — deadlines to be met, assignments to be completed, financial burdens that weigh upon us without any hope of remission, the boredom of the suburban housewife's daily drudgery. Our hospitals are filled with the victims of stress, while our sports fields abound with those who are constructively channelling this pressure. A certain amount of stress is necessary for all of us if we are to function efficiently and with enthusiasm and vitality. As Yerkes has shown, there is a definite relationship between stress and efficiency. The positive effects are evident until, at a certain point, a level is reached where inefficiency results. This so-called stress threshold differs for each one according to personality and physiological make-up. Once it is reached, not only does performance decline, but if the pressure continues it will lead to a variety of illnesses.

Stress, as defined by Peter Tyrer, 'is the reaction of the mind and body to change',[1] whether it be agreeable or disagreeable, desired or feared. When one is able to adapt well to change, the stress can add to proficiency. When the powers of adaptation fail, effectiveness is diminished until finally there is a breakdown in both mental and physical health.

Stress then can be a constructive and energising force leading to an enthusiastic and wholehearted involvement, or it can become destructive, causing a variety of emotional reactions, for instance anxiety or anger, with harmful physical effects. Anything from within or from the world around us which evokes this type of response is called a stressor.

Mid-life is a time of particular vulnerability to such stressors because of the deep psychological changes taking place. It is a time, too, when greater pressure comes from added responsibilities or other claims on our energies. A variety of emotional, psychological, intellectual, physical, social and spiritual factors can be identified which give rise to this additional pressure in the mid years.

Emotional factors

An emotional instability often characterises this time of life. There can be excessive worry over trifles or various fears unknown in earlier years. For the first time the sudden appearance of a mouse may alarm us out of all proportion, or we may be afraid to enter an empty house alone. The added demands of our position in society can bring with it a host of what might be called anticipatory fears, anxiety as to how to cope with an interview, give a lecture or present oneself at an official engagement. Then there are all those insistent minor worries, free-floating fears, whose cause we do not know. For the most part these spring from an underlying sense of inferiority and a persistent attitude of self-doubt. Worry about caring for ageing parents, of providing for the extra demands of adolescent children, of taking on new responsibilities in work or profession can also overwhelm the mid-lifer.

A further emotional stressor common at this time is guilt. We feel guilty as we look back at the past, or because we cannot cope in meeting the emotional and other demands of parents or relatives who have become dependent in their old age. This sense of guilt, like all other emotions, is an important indicator that something is not as right as we would like. Having registered that message it is vital to let go of the sense of culpability, not hold on to it, feeling, in some strange way, that to be guilty is to compensate for past mistakes. Unrelinquished, this emotion can become one of the most detrimental stressors.

Anger, too, is a significant cause of stress at this stage, as at other times in life — so important that we shall examine it separately in a later section. The earlier repression of many emotions and desires can also produce a hidden stress which can be highly damaging if not dealt with in this second half of life. This, too, will be looked at later on.

Psychological factors

Low self-esteem is characteristic of the middle years and becomes one of the most striking psychological stressors. We experience the disintegration of our former self-image, which so often takes place during the mid-life crisis, as an attack on our self-worth. Self-confidence then takes a battering. Personality types will be affected in different ways according to their psychological make-up. For the naturally ambitious person, the Type A personality, the pressures of mid-life present serious challenges to his or her well-being, but these, however, are not as marked for the Type B, the more placid personality. There is a range of personality types beyond these two, and each reacts to stressors in a characteristic fashion. The anxious personality is highly prone to excessive stress during these years as emotional changes lead to exaggeration of anxiety. The dependent person is constantly threatened by a changing self-image and the fear that others may no longer appreciate him or her. Some personality types tend to become excessively fussy, others to be suspicious or overly demanding and these all meet added strain from the emotional or physical changes of mid-life. The more carefree personality is less affected on the whole by the normal stressors of this time of life.

Intellectual and social factors

Intellectual stressors abound in the decisions and choices involved in increasing responsibility in career or family matters. The demands made by a business world which deals more readily in tens of millions than in thousands, can weigh heavily upon those in managerial positions today. One false move, or one inconsidered step, can lead to the rapid loss of a business built up over years. Stress meets us at every turn. Because of the irascibility brought on by these added professional concerns, relationships can suffer both within and beyond the home. It is no wonder, then, that breakdowns in communication between spouses or partners, or with teenage children commonly occur and give rise to a sense of alienation and loneliness. Many, also, still hold on to unrealistic goals and continue to strive for the unattainable to the detriment of both their health and family, or other relationships.

Physical factors

A deterioration in physical health, especially for men, can become a serious stressor during mid-life. It is a recognised fact that men suffer from ill-health more than women do at this time. The prospect, or actuality, of a severe illness brings with it not only incapacity but also an additional burden of apprehension for the future and anxiety about what is happening at work or in the home. Added to this is the concern over ensuing financial difficulties. Sometimes in an effort to relieve mounting stress, further stressors, perhaps alcohol, caffeine or nicotine, are taken and do no more than complicate the condition. Financial pressures can arise as well from the increasing demands of adolescent children, or perhaps from expectations to entertain in a way appropriate to a new professional role. The need for frequent travel as the result of promotion at this time can be an added stressor for the business man or woman.

The physiology of stress

To understand the effects of stress on the body it is necessary to understand how we react physiologically to any stressor. Imagine someone lying quietly on the beach, basking in the sun, lulled by the sound of the sea and feeling utterly relaxed. Then suddenly a cry for help from the surf shatters the peace. Immediately the body is geared for action. The adrenal glands pour adrenalin into the system. The person leaps to his or her feet, eyes wide open, pupils dilated for maximum vision and senses alert. The blood flows from the digestive system to the muscles which tense up ready for prompt action, breathing is shallow and the heart beat rapid. Now aroused, the individual is prepared to rush to the rescue. If, however, all is well and it was only a false alarm, the sunbathing is resumed and slowly the body returns to balance as the adrenalin and other chemicals drain out of the bloodstream. In the space of a few minutes the whole system has been geared to action and returned again to relaxation.

The autonomic nervous system directs this change in bodily responses and is distinct from the central nervous system which governs voluntary action. It controls the movements of the blood vessel walls, the gastro-intestinal system, the dilatation of the tiny air passages in the lungs and the many movements in our bodies of which we are not even aware. This system consists of two parts, the sympathetic and the parasympathetic systems. When the body is under the influence of the latter, it is relaxed and calm. Its function is to bring about the digestion and storage of food and to maintain the body in a balanced state and it is sometimes referred to as the 'rest and digest' system. If action is needed, the sympathetic, 'the fight or flight', system takes over. Under its influence a mixture of chemicals including adrenalin, norepinephrine and finally — if stress continues — cortisone, are released into the bloodstream to prepare the body for exertion and to maintain it in action. When these chemicals remain in the blood for a prolonged period the level of cholesterol rises. Once the body relaxes and the parasympathetic system has resumed control, these chemicals are no longer produced and gradually disappear from the bloodstream. However, if they remain in the blood for a prolonged period as a result of continued sympathetic stimulation, an adverse effect on various organs soon occurs.

It is obvious that anyone living a normal healthy life will fluctuate between being under the influence of the sympathetic and parasympathetic system according to need. For someone, however, who is under constant stress the sympathetic system remains in control and the build up of potentially harmful chemicals becomes dangerously high.

The effect of cholesterol on the small coronary vessels of the heart is well-known. Less known is the fact that norepinephrine can give rise to constriction of small vessels and also clotting of the blood. Blood pressure is raised as a result of the presence of both of these compounds. For this reason coronary occlusion or other heart disease and strokes are frequently closely linked with stress.

Cortisone, when present in the bloodstream for a prolonged time, tends to suppress the formation of lymphocytes, the white blood cells which are the body's defence against viral and bacterial infection. It is now generally recognised that certain cancers may be viral in origin. The effect of the prolonged presence of a high level of these chemicals in the blood brings about a reaction of exhaustion. Some body cells simply die, not infrequently those of the lining of the duodenum, the first section of the small intestine, or of the stomach wall. When this occurs the acid of the gastric juice erodes the lining, and a gastric, duodenal or peptic ulcer is formed. Other gastro-intestinal effects of prolonged stress are indigestion, spasm of the colon with distension above the constricted area and severe pain, colitis and a variety of associated disorders.

Constant muscular tension from sustained stress gives rise to neck, chest and back pains, headache and respiratory disorders. Tension may also be the cause of menstrual disturbances, skin rashes and allergies. Ailments such as the nagging pain of a developing duodenal ulcer, or constant headaches, are often the first indications of excessive stress.

Unlike tension, stress is not felt as a physical sensation, so it is possible to be considerably stressed without being aware of it. It is critical, then, that we listen to our bodies for these messages of unhealthy pressure before harm is done.

Coping with stress

Relaxation, the outcome of parasympathetic activity, is incompatible with stress. Anything, therefore, which is relaxing will relieve its immediate effects and bring the body back into a healthy balance. It is often not possible to eliminate all harmful stress from living, but periods of relaxation in stressful situations will prevent a damaging build-up of the effects of prolonged sympathetic stimulation. Everyone knows what is most relaxing for him- or herself and this differs for each one. Breathing exercises have the advantage of guaranteeing an adequate oxygen supply, for oxygen lack is a direct cause of anxiety and tension. These exercises, together with finding a quiet place in our minds or imagination, where we can escape for five or ten minutes, can be a splendid means of relaxing in the midst of a busy day. To leave behind the pressures of work and escape for a short break into a peaceful country scene or to walk along the seashore in fantasy can relieve stress and renew jaded energy. The techniques of t'ai chi, the exercises of yoga or transcendental meditation, for example, also provide an excellent means of slowing down the pace of a high-pressured life-style. Some find jogging, walking, swimming or gardening profitable as well as enjoyable.

It is often necessary to look at self-imposed pressures, expectations or unreal ambitions that we have. An attitude that is constantly blaming or worrying might well be changed to one that seeks out the positive aspects of a situation. For example, even if we have missed the bus to work, no one is helped by spending the next twenty minutes worrying over the consequences. If instead we look for the positive outcome — that this gives us an extra twenty minutes to sit and read or knit or simply to reflect — we will arrive at work, late certainly, but much healthier. What could have become a treadmill of anxiety has been transformed into a period of relaxation.

An excellent task for many is to make a pie graph, a simple circle drawn on paper. Then, just as a pie is cut up, the graph is divided into segments according to how the day, the week, or perhaps the year, is spent. How much time is allocated to recreation, to work, to socialising? To see a picture such as this can be a helpful way of recognising the need to restructure one's life: to search for a novel or detective story for light reading, to take up some new sport or recreative pastime, or to spend time simply enjoying the beauties of nature. There will always be unfinished business in life. To learn to abandon the compulsion to complete everything before taking a break will lead to a far healthier and happier life.

Burnout

For years there has been talk of burnout, countrysides burnt out, homes and cities completely destroyed by fire. Motors and engines have been burning out since they were first invented, but it is only since the early 1970s that this term has been applied to a human condition. We, like the machines we operate, can burn out, give up in a state of complete exhaustion.

This phenomenon, though stress-related, is not the same as stress. It follows a well-defined pattern, as was pointed out by Dr Edelwich in 1974, and is accompanied by a loss of energy and purpose.

The first signs of burnout are a lessening of the customary interest and involvement in the work in hand, a dulling of enthusiasm and with it a depletion of energy. Boredom sets in. Accustomed occupations become tedious and there is a sense of being caught in a rut. In the words of a devoted worker for the disabled: 'I am beginning to feel afraid. A deep change seems to be going on inside me and I don't know what is happening. Once I loved my job and really knew I was helping people. I still do in a way, but I'm starting to be bored and restless and am no longer satisfied in the way I was before.' She was experiencing the first symptoms of burnout. A common reaction to this situation is to feel unproductive and, therefore, guilty. So one works harder and for longer hours to compensate, but this merely complicates the condition.

Self-esteem suffers and a state of frustration and hopelessness ensues. The job itself is blamed for the inability to cope and its suitability is questioned. Finally, apathy sets in. The welfare of those ministered to or for whom one works is no longer a concern. Sarcasm, cynicism or even a type of protective arrogance may creep into dealings with others. With an increasingly negative approach, the person becomes disillusioned and resentful, sinking into a persistent state of depression. This is burnout. One can be in varying stages of the condition for an indefinite period. Some live most of their lives in a state of semi-burnout.

Not only does work or ministry suffer, but the symptoms of burnout are carried into the home and social life. The individual in burnout becomes a dull and apathetic companion. Sleep is elusive, leaving one habitually tired and without energy. Occasionally, uncharacteristic outbursts of anger, or atypically tactless remarks, surprise and disconcert relatives or friends. Many of the same somatic symptoms that characterise stress develop: loss of appetite, gastro-intestinal disorders or headaches. Sleep, when it comes, does not seem to refresh or revitalise. There is an incessant feeling of tiredness or exhaustion. A changing attitude colours grey a world which once was full of challenge and excitement.

Burnout is a condition which affects men and women equally, especially those in the helping professions. Ministers, social workers, teachers, those in the counselling or medical professions are particularly prone to this phenomenon. The reason for this lies both with the persons involved and those for whom they work. Those who feel called to devote themselves in these areas are, for the most part, strongly motivated with high ideals as to the outcome they seek. They are dedicated to the welfare of others and are frequently frustrated at the failure of their efforts to achieve the relief or the cure they had anticipated. Even when they do succeed in one area there is a never-ending call for their services and the task ahead seems endless. The emotional demands made by this type of service can be excessive and more often than not fail to be balanced by satisfying feedback. Mitchell suggests that it is this non-reciprocity between consultant and client which is the root cause of burnout.[2] A constant giving without adequate return proves in the long run to be emotionally draining and will lead to frustration and a depletion of personal resources. All have need of a sense of satisfaction or success, if they are to keep vitally involved in a way that is life-giving to clients, patients or pupils as well as to themselves.

To avoid burnout means to employ ways that will

help to build up energy rather than constantly deplete it. John Sanford points out that anything that calls forth our creative powers will be re-energising.[3] One important area of creativity is to be found in our relationships with friends other than professional colleagues. Dr Glasser, the founder of Reality Therapy, also lists this as one of the ingredients he prescribes for the prevention of burnout. He speaks of the need for 'a requisite daily portion of love'. This, together with sufficient fun and relaxation, an adequate dose of success in work, and the ability to set limits on the demands made on oneself, is his prescription for an antidote to burnout.

Remaining open to new suggestions, trying novel ways of production, experimenting with fresh methods of performing customary tasks, be they as small as finding a new recipe or fishing spot, all keep us alert and open to change. The teacher who encourages pupil participation in original ways is less likely to suffer burnout. The nurse who does not allow herself to be caught in a daily routine but tries to bring variety to her own and her patients' lives, will be energised rather than drained by her profession. Woodwork, crafts or dabbling in art or music can all be stimulating.

Due heed should also be given to time out in order to restore energy. Short breaks just to sit and be in a busy day, or to dip into an interesting novel can rekindle vigour. It is difficult to say 'no' to a request which would cut across this necessary period of relaxation and recuperation. But unless we can put aside adequate space to replenish resources, to dissociate from the pressures of normal routines and immerse ourselves deeply in a fresh and stimulating environment, we not only do harm to ourselves but have little of worth to offer others.

Burnout is not so much a problem involving work, as one of giving insufficient time to re-creative pastimes and enjoyments, of failing to come to terms with the fact that there will always be unfinished business or imperfection in our day and of realising that life was never intended to be a constant treadmill of activity, but rather a balance between a giving of ourselves, and a replenishment of our resources.

♦ ♦ ♦

Chapter • 7

UNDERSTANDING ANGER

Of all the emotions perhaps anger is the most misunderstood and maligned. Society on the whole regards it with a great deal of uncertainty; some rush in encouraging a variety of aggressive behaviours, while others tend to ignore its significance altogether. For those in the second half of life the understanding of anger assumes a particular importance. Not only are emotions less stable in the early part of mid-life, but with the expansion of consciousness at this stage of life, much vexation and resentment that was repressed in early years begins to surface, or to make its presence felt in various ways.

Anger is a normal, healthy and valuable emotion. It is an intrinsic part of human nature and should be respected as such, for it plays an important role in every healthy life. One of the most powerful of all the emotions, it can be used creatively or misused in a destructive fashion. Once aroused it liberates considerable energy which can well be directed into constructive enterprises, like working to achieve a more just society, when it is the injustices that have given rise to our indignation.

At other times the same energy, when not directed into positive channels, can wreak havoc. This happens when we lose mastery of our actions, giving over the control to the emotion itself. It is especially the case when anger has been allowed to build up, has not been recognised and expressed, until it reaches major proportions. These irate outbursts or explosions can be too strong for rational control and the person is more often than not, quite unaware of how damaging the resulting behaviour may be. We all know the effect this has on the recipient, who may be responsible simply for the 'last straw' that causes an eruption like that of Vesuvius. It can be a traumatic and crushing experience, making it extremely difficult to recover from or to forget such an explosion. At the same time, with the release of built up tension, the angry person feels a sense of relief and has very little idea of how deeply affected the other may be.

The extremely irascible who can no longer control the expression of their indignation often wonder why others fear them. They seem oblivious to the damage an outburst of this kind can do to a relationship. I have frequently had these people say to me: 'I can't understand why it is so difficult to find any real friends. I make advances to others, but they seem afraid to let me come close to them.' There is in most people a real fear of the unmitigated anger of another. No wonder they are apprehensive about moving into a close relationship with such an individual. On the other hand, anger when expressed appropriately, can have a very beneficial effect on any honest friendship. It leads to a clearing of the air and allows for greater understanding and empathy between friends.

Much of the misunderstanding surrounding this emotion comes from the misperception that it is not right to be angry. It is the outcome of anger which incites to destructive behaviour towards oneself or others that involves morality. In itself anger is morally neutral, as are all the emotions. It is what it may lead to that can become morally wrong. When it was listed among the 'capital' sins it was not the emotion which was being condemned as immoral. The word 'capital' derives from the Latin 'caput', the head or source of action. Anger, a spontaneous emotion outside the domain of morality, is, however, acknowledged to be a major source of behaviour which can readily become immoral.

Because, also, some expressions of anger on the part of a child can be experienced as painful or undesirable by the adult, many children receive a message early in life that the anger itself is wrong, and is not acceptable. It is difficult for the young child to distinguish between the emotion and the action by which he or she chooses to express it. So it is the anger, rather than the action, that appears wrong. All these communications which have been picked up directly or indirectly throughout life can lead to a refusal to recognise anger when it is present, to deny or repress it.

Rather, it should be perceived as a valuable resource in living for all of us. It is a normal reaction which indicates that some harm to our person or our interests is pending or has occurred. Anything which assails self-esteem, diminishes self-worth, or harms us in any respect, will elicit this particular emotion. It can been seen, then, as a messenger that alerts us to the fact that our welfare is under threat in some way. Even the newborn baby can experience real rage if its basic needs remain unmet. Its cries, flushed face and tightly clenched fists are clear evidence of this.

It is not always easy to recognise that we are angry, especially if we are not accustomed to registering our feelings. Anger can easily be camouflaged as 'being upset', 'hurt' or 'anxious'. A powerful emotional stressor, it brings the body under the influence of the sympathetic nervous system with the physiological reactions looked at earlier. When we are aware of these changes in the body, tenseness or tightness, burning face or ears, it is essential to identify the cause and be able to own it. To name and admit our anger gives the freedom necessary to choose a healthy way in which to express it. When we are unaware of what is happening, the anger often takes over and reveals itself in ways beyond our control. Once aware of emotional arousal, we will recognise the cause as anger if we know we are being belittled or frustrated in some way. This is the message it always brings: something is blocking legitimate needs or desires or is in some other way disparaging either us or those whose welfare concerns us.

As shown on the diagram (see page 93), this blocking is called a frustration and will arise from the behaviour of an individual or even at times from an inanimate object, a door that always sticks or a car that will not start. The normal response to this sort of a frustration is the emotion of anger. Once recognised, this leaves a choice of what we wish to do as a result. If we ignore the feeling or fail to give any expression to it, its effects will continue even when it is banished to unconsciousness. Since it is a stressor, it will have a physiological effect which will be damaging to the body in various ways. Three options then are open: to choose to give some overt expression to anger; to suppress it, that is recognise its presence but decide to put it aside for the moment and concentrate on something else; or, finally, to repress it. This implies that as

The pattern of anger

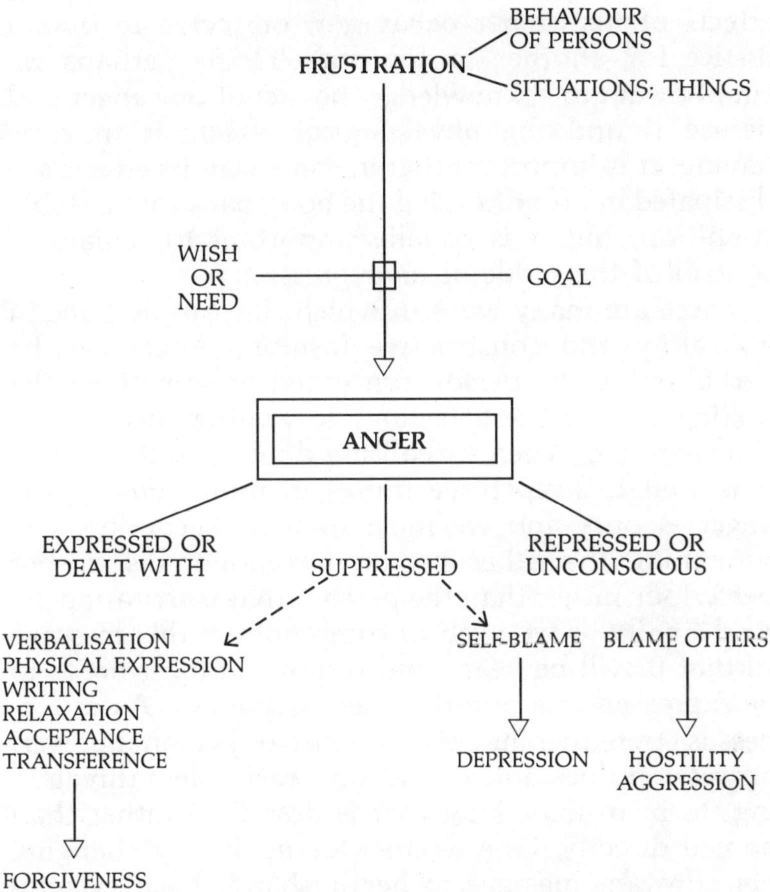

Figure 7.1

the result of an earlier decision not to accept this feeling, we are not even conscious of its presence. The anger simply remains below the level of consciousness and is added to the storehouse of previously unrecognised and unexpressed emotions.

If we decide to give expression to the feeling, there is a choice between various ways of acting. What is chosen will depend on the outcome desired. Are we seeking revenge, wanting the other to be aware of the effects of his or her behaviour, or trying to obtain justice for another or for oneself? Or perhaps we simply want to acknowledge the fact of our anger and defuse it and the physiological effects it may be having. It is important that in some way its effects are dissipated in order to bring the body back into a stable condition, but it is equally important to remain in control of the mode of its expression.

There are many ways in which this can be done in a healthy and constructive fashion. Anger can be verbalised to the person concerned or sometimes the talking out of these feelings to another can give a similar relief. When verbalising directly to the person it is well to keep three things in mind. Firstly, the anger is ours and we must own it. Secondly, it is something the other person has done, his or her behaviour rather than the person, that is irritating us. And finally, if we wish to communicate this message so that it will be heard and responded to, it needs to be expressed in a non-threatening manner. Assertiveness is strengthening, gives a sense of personal power, aggression does not. It is always easier, less threatening, to hear something that is described rather than named directly. One woman learnt this by changing her constant message to her husband. Each evening that he came in aggressively looking for a meal that was not yet ready, she would retort with something like: 'You make me wild stamping in here demanding a meal when it isn't cooked yet.' When she tried instead: 'I really do get angry when you keep expecting to find the meal on the table, even though you can see it isn't cooked yet', he began then to see his own irrationality and consequently his way of acting changed.

Some type of physical expression can also give relief from the stress of anger. It is true that if not used correctly this can result in an increase rather than a lessening of the emotion. When such expression leads to a sense of personal worth, or trust in our own strength, it can be a valuable way of 'letting go' rather than 'storing up' our feelings. If it becomes a way of asserting ourselves to promote and strengthen the self-esteem which has been damaged, it can be a mature and useful method of overcoming any possible harm.

Writing, too, can achieve the same end. To write either in letter or dialogue form helps to explore the depths of the indignation and to get in touch with its effects on us. One precaution is necessary here. It is rarely a wise thing to send the letter which gives vent to these first impulses. Time is required before what really needs to be communicated can be expressed in a way that is not too emotionally charged. The first letter is often best assigned to the wastepaper bin, while the second will carry a more rational message.

If the choice is simply to dissipate feelings of anger so that we are freed in body and mind of the disturbing effects of this arousal, there are many options open. Anything that is calming or relaxing, will have the desired effect.

It is possible too to come to terms with these feelings once we have registered them; to know that even though what is happening may be frustrating, it is little enough compared with the burden carried by some.

It can also happen that when we review situations which once caused bitter indignation, quite a different interpretation of the incident comes to mind. This is often the case with childhood traumas or misunderstandings when seen again through adult eyes. The situation, reappraised in this way, loses it original threat and we recognise the stress under which parents perhaps laboured or some other moderating factor. The anger which may have been stored for years is then dissipated as acceptance comes with this new understanding.

There are some situations, however, which do not allow for the immediate expression of annoyance. In these cases, it may be necessary to acknowledge the feelings and then consciously put them aside to be resolved at an appropriate time later. The very diversion of concentration and energy to another area may be sufficient to dispel the emotional disturbance or it may be necessary later to use methods, like those already mentioned, to restore equilibrium.

The danger lies in a non-recognition of anger, a failing to allow ourselves even to register it, so that it moves directly into the unconscious and remains active there, seeping out in a multitude of different ways.

To repress an emotion in this way leads to a variety of behavioural problems whose source may be difficult to identify. Repressed anger can be turned inwards, resulting in a high level of anxiety, with a tendency to self-blame and self-hatred. This invariably leads to depression with all the symptoms which accompany it. It is one of the most common causes of depression in all those I have had in therapy. Many are even unaware of their depression, having become so accustomed to feeling as they do. They have acquired an at-homeness with their negative feelings, their inability to make decisions or their powerlessness to get themselves going. One woman of fifty became aware of her depression only on reading her journal of the past year and being struck by the number of entries which spoke of the lack of desire to continue living. Surely, she thought, that was not what life was meant to be about, yet this was the way she had felt since childhood. Therapy helped her to uncover the cause of much of her anger, repressed because she had felt she could not admit to it in her early days at school. When this was faced her depression quickly lifted.

We may, on the other hand, unconsciously choose to turn the force of repressed anger outwards. This gives rise to an attitude of hostility, of blaming others, of aggressiveness and, what is perhaps more difficult to recognise and deal with, passive-aggressiveness. This refers to the seeping out of anger in a twisted fashion. Passive-aggressives tend to clothe their negativity with a thin veneer of the positive. Their statements so often include a 'but': 'That's a wonderful idea, but do you really think you could carry it through?' The recipient of such a remark immediately feels in some way sabotaged. Other distorted expressions of repressed anger are found in disturbances of weight through compensatory over-eating or starvation, disorders in sleep patterns, and many psychosomatic illnesses.

How can the presence of this type of repression be recognised? Firstly, we may become aware that one or other of the above descriptions seems to fit well. Feelings of guilt or of hurt can be another indication, or tears that are constantly close to the surface. The tendency not to notice someone or to be unaware of his or her needs, or the propensity to forget to do what one particular person has asked can all be indicators that there is repressed indignation towards that person. All the physical and physiological disabilities already discussed in the chapter on stress may also be caused by this particular stressor: ulcers, skin disorders, allergies, and so on.

When any powerful emotion, such as fear or anger,

is repressed it tends to block many of the weaker ones, thus leading to an emotional crippling and an alienation from our true feelings. After freeing up an enormous weight of repressed fear and anger a professional woman declared that she found herself seeing things differently. When asked in what way, she replied that now when she looked at something beautiful in nature or at someone in distress, she could sense it 'right through her being'. Before it had always been somehow 'outside' of her.

Once aware of the presence of repressed anger it is essential to try, often with the assistance of a psychotherapist or counsellor, to bring it to consciousness so that it is possible to acknowledge and own it. It can then be dealt with in the ways already suggested. But a truly Christian resolution is not complete until there is forgiveness for those responsible for the harm done. In the words of Hannah Arendt: 'Forgiveness is an eminently personal affair in which *what* was done is forgiven for the sake of *who* did it.'[1] Forgiveness may not necessarily be felt, but if it is truly in the will then pardon has been given.

One important group of people who are rarely conscious of how angry they are in reality are those who are sometimes called the 'pleasers' of society. They are the people who are always trying to satisfy others, to live up to their expectations, to keep the peace at any cost. Unknowingly, they are constantly depriving themselves of the freedom to express their own needs and desires and, in consequence, are continually depreciating themselves. Charles Schwab once said: 'A man who trims himself to suit everyone will soon whittle himself away.'[2]

Many perfectionists also harbour deep stores of anger, often towards themselves, because they are never able to reach the high standards they have set.

There is a reluctance, too, to admit to being angry as this is seen as an imperfection. In consequence the emotion is repressed. There are also a large number of women and men who have suffered deprivation of their basic needs in early life, or perhaps of other needs in more recent years. It is this constant frustration which gives rise to an anger of which they may be completely unaware.

The psychiatrist, Conrad Baars, is convinced of the importance of this area of emotional crippling when he writes: 'The widespread repression of anger in our society deserves serious study since its consequences are many and varied, more so than those of the repression of sexual feelings ever were.' But he warns: 'An accurate understanding of ... anger as well as of the mechanism of repression is an absolute must ... Without this understanding pop-psychology, in its attempts to attack the prevailing ignorance about anger and aggression, threatens to create new psychic disorders.'[3]

Anger, also, often conceals some other underlying feeling, perhaps of fear or helplessness. In the case of children who have been abused there can be a level of deep sadness which can only be released when the attendant anger is faced and dealt with. One man, in recalling being belittled and laughed at as a small child by his father, discovered the depth of hurt and anger within him. When he allowed himself to stay with this for a while he became filled with a profound sense of sadness and tears began to flow for the first time in his life. This feeling of sadness remained with him over several days until both the anger and sorrow were released.

Once there is some understanding of how this emotion is aroused, it becomes possible to modify its intensity. Frustration can be lessened by our being more realistic in our expectations and desires. We can discover different ways of moving towards objectives or satisfying needs, and come to a deeper sensitivity to the problems facing those whose actions irritate us.

The energy produced by anger can be channelled into many constructive activities. It was the indignation engendered by seeing a family driven onto the streets by a grasping landlord that inspired a young businessman to initiate an investigation into the rights of the poor. This resulted in the establishment of a place of refuge for the homeless.

Dr Baars tells the story of how anger was 'a life-saving factor' for him during two years of imprisonment in the Nazi concentration camp of Buchenwald. Of the one thousand prisoners sent to the camp with him only six survived to see the liberation led by General Patton. 'Next to my faith in God, it was my constant anger at the Nazis for having deprived me of my liberty, and their inhuman treatment of their prisoners, that stimulated my determination to survive and to deny them the satisfaction of seeing me die. My anger ... provided me with energy to survive hard labour, a starvation diet and other hardships. Though I could never display it in any form, neither did I repress it. It was constantly directed by my reason which told me that to become outwardly angry at my captors would mean certain death. Prayer and anger allowed me to see the hour of liberation...'[4]

In both these cases the anger could be fruitfully kept alive and nurtured since its outcome was life-giving or led to a situation where basic rights were respected. It remained the motivating force providing both the strength and energy to carry on in such situations.

Before finishing this topic, it might be well to look for a moment at an area of profound chagrin, hurt and resentment in our society. The cultural devaluation of women and their exploitation has been a source of much deep-seated, though often unrecognised, anger. In the words of Margaret Brennan: 'Women, like the earth, have been a symbol of that which can be objectified, dominated, controlled, raped, plundered and devalued.'[5] In retaliation to this devaluation women have at times reciprocated in ways unhelpful both to themselves and to those who, perhaps unwittingly, disparage them. Because such expressions have proved threatening to others, they have led to further opposition and little real understanding or support. Behind this anger, and often completely obscured by it, lies a profound sense of sadness that what women have to offer to the church, the professions and society in general is considered, in some way, second class. In these situations women often find themselves patronised, put down or made to feel unsure of their own worth. Their anger cannot be by-passed but once entered into and integrated it may well lead to a meaningful and constructive expression. For 'anger is no final resting place'.[6]

In the case of many women it has become the wellspring of creative energy that is life-giving in its expression of the feminine spirit in a male-dominated culture. The discovery that 'the old rage is love and power'[7] can strengthen women for that most female of all tasks, to bring healing and new life. In this transformation of the power of anger lies the promise of the future recognition of women's strength and wisdom and the part they both must play in the society of the future.

♦ ♦ ♦

Chapter • 8

DEVELOPMENT AND INTEGRATION OF SEXUALITY

We belong to a long tradition of expressed appreciation of the mystery and wonder of sexuality but one which, at the same time, seems filled with fear and apprehension of this singular gift. In the first book of the bible we read that God created humankind in the image of himself, man and woman he created them, and 'God saw all that he had made and indeed it was very good.' (Genesis 1:31) This is the way the early Israelites understood the dignity of both women and men, and the sacredness of their being formed in the likeness of their Maker.

When St Irenaeus, in the second century, declared that 'the glory of God is humankind fully alive', he was calling on the early Christians to understand that their humanness in its entirety was what God looked for in them, not some form of angelism. To be human on every level and not to reject or fear their human impulses; to be 'fully alive', spiritually, physically, intellectually, sexually; only in this manner could they glorify God in the way that he desired.

In a recent article published in *Sojourner*, Richard Rohr of the New Jerusalem Community in the USA wrote, 'I am convinced that our sexual lives are the most universally damaged part of our human nature.' There are a vast number of priests, psychiatrists, counsellors and ordinary men and women in the street who would very readily agree with him. Instead of appreciating and coming to understand our sexuality, we have tended to be suspicious of it or to over-react against the restraints of an earlier period. In an age that is 'sexually liberated', many seem to have lost all sense of true freedom in this area and have become enslaved to one aspect of their sexuality, the genital. To be truly liberated from the misunderstanding and fears that have surrounded this area of human nature means first to comprehend sexuality in a holistic sense, and to have an integral view of the meaning of being a sexual person.

Sexuality is not something limited to one part of the body. It permeates the whole of our being. It is the vehicle of reaching out to others, socialising and perhaps becoming intimate with them. Through a bodily presence we are acceptable to others in ways that are welcoming, tender and warm. This relatedness with them is rooted in our sexuality and can only be freely expressed when we are 'at home' with ourselves.

To appreciate sexuality implies an understanding of the modes of its expression. It denotes, too, the ability to develop each of these so as to integrate them into the personality. These aspects are often referred to as primary, affective and genital sexuality, and together form an integral part of our wholeness as human persons. These three elements are inextricably intertwined and, though separate, function in unison to bring harmony and fulfilment to our lives.

Although there is a bisexuality in human beings, each is primarily either woman or man. Every cell in the body gives evidence of this in the matching of its chromosones, XX in the woman, XY in the man. This is manifest, not only in the body structure, but also in the many ways we function psychologically, spiritually, or socially. Primary sexuality refers to the maleness or femaleness that predominates in each person and out of which that person operates. Do we ever pause to ask ourselves are we contented, even proud, to be man or woman? Have we really accepted our primary sexuality and enjoyed our masculinity or femininity?

To be comfortable with this dimension of sexuality as evidenced in our bodies is a necessary step to full individuation. To accept, respect and appreciate the body is an important part of coming to a wholeness. Failing to do so results in a stunted response to life and is reflected in the way we view others and the world around us. It is only too easy to acquire the habit of rejecting parts of our person; hands because they are too big, legs which are unshapely, breasts that seem too small. Until the whole is owned and accepted as it is and appreciated because it is part of our totality, there will be a lack of full development. Some maintain that it is easier for women to accept their bodies in this way than it is for men.

It is the body that will give the first indication of ill health, of renewed energy, or the need for a celebration of life. As Jim Zullo assures us: 'The body never lies.' If we listen to our headaches, our backaches or stomachaches and respond to the obvious indication there, then life will be much healthier. If we can hear the messages of pleasure or elation and give expression to them, living will become a far more joyful experience.

Being attentive to the body, listening to its communication of stress, of joy, of pain, moves one to an awareness and self-knowledge without which there can be no true self-actualisation.

It would seem also that there are some basic differences in the ways men and women function and perceive reality. We have already looked at how much this may depend on cultural expectations and how much is inherent. It is, however, widely agreed that 'a woman's existence tends to be centred, whole and caring, whereas a man's inclines to be differentiated, compartmentalised and task-oriented'.[1] Women, in their relating, usually look more for love than genital expression, more for an intimacy of oneness of spirit with the other. They have deep affective needs and long to be touched, held and re-assured. Men are more protective, more conscious of their need to provide for others. They, on the whole, seem to value genital expression in a relationship more highly than do women.

During the years of mid-life both men and women may find a change taking place as they integrate more and more of the opposite sex characteristics of the anima or animus, becoming more androgynous. This enrichment of sexuality empowers the man to become increasingly centred, tender and loving in his relating, as the woman grows more sure of herself and freer in the expression of her needs.

The body, too, is changing as a result of alterations in hormonal levels, and the early signs of ageing begin to make their appearance. It is not always easy to welcome the greying or receding hair-line, eyes that can no longer see to read the small print and a sometimes rapidly expanding waistline. One of the challenges of mid-life for many is to come to terms with these indications of maturing age as revealed through this bodily 'trans-figuration'.

Affective sexuality

The affective dimension of sexuality has the greatest influence on our growth to full maturity and integration. When Maslow spoke of the fundamental needs which must be met in any human person on the journey to self-actualisation, he described as basic, not that of genital sexuality, but rather that of a felt relationship with some other human being. We are far more aware now of the necessity for affirmation and love from infancy if a child is to develop into a person who can both give and receive love in later life. If love is absent, or unfelt, in these early years, it is not possible for the affective element of sexuality to mature fully. Moreover, the warm and tender feelings which should be there to nurture the next generation are missing. This lack can be passed through one generation to the next. An unloved child, or one who has not felt affirmed, will become a mother or a father incapable of expressing love in her or his turn. So the cycle prolongs itself until special care is given to overcome the problem.

All the loving, tender and warm feelings, emotions or moods which incline to intimacy or closeness with another have their source in this dimension of sexuality. Their growth depends on the circumstances of one's upbringing.

In *The Growth of Love and Sex*, Jack Dominian traces the development of affective sexuality from the time in infancy when the foundations of love and sex are laid through the relationship with the mother.

Feelings of acceptance and tenderness are communicated to the infant especially through the sense of touch, but also through the sight of the mother's face and the sound of her voice. This initial bonding in love 'becomes the pattern for attachment later on with friends, lovers and spouses'.[2] As children advance through Erikson's stages they come to a sense of independence or autonomy and an ability to separate from the parent. When this is encouraged gently by the parent, trust and a healthy love of self grow within the child. It becomes able to internalise the image of the mother and to maintain feelings of affection and warmth towards her even in her absence.

The initiative crisis occurs as the four-to-five-year-old struggles with the need, in the boy, to find identity with his father apart from his mother, Freud's oedipal complex, and in the little girl to give up her sexual (non-genital) attraction towards her father to identify with her mother, the electra complex. During this period children need constant affirmation and love if they are to consolidate a positive image of themselves as loveable people. Failure on the part of parents to provide this affectionate and affirming environment for the child results in insecurity, self-doubt, fear and sometimes complete withdrawal.

The school-age child learns to extend the boundaries of love and friendship to embrace a community of both adults and other children, to make allowance for others and to treat them with concern and justice. Loyalty to friends, especially those of the same sex, grows as the young person reaches adolescence. Strong feelings of infatuation with members of the opposite sex are common. At times a member of the same sex or a much older person can be the object of these feelings. The adolescent's powers of loving are strengthened and deepened by these encounters which are normally short-lived and often involve the combination of genital arousal.

It is at this time, too, that homosexual attraction may predominate, especially in environments which encourage it, for example single-sexed boarding establishments. This may give way to heterosexual preference as opportunities to mix with members of the opposite sex become more readily available. As the adolescent struggles to find his or her identity, homosexual feelings can be as strong and as erotic as heterosexual ones. There is nothing abnormal in this. It is not until the mid-twenties that a person clearly recognises his or her true sexual orientation through observing over time the direction of attraction, affection and responsiveness. Homosexuality becomes evident, as a rule, in the area of affective sexuality rather than genital.

Love blossoms as the young adult is drawn to a relationship of intimacy with another. This is normally rooted in a strong affective attraction which is frequently accompanied by genital excitation and desire.

At mid-life and throughout the later years generative strivings are based in our affective sexuality as growing concern and care for others motivates activities. There is a call, too, to deeper intimacy both with the emerging Self and with others. This is rooted in the new level of personality integration, which brings with it a freedom to love more selflessly and to give more freely in service.

The area of affective sexuality is one which all are called to develop whether they be married or celibate, that is unmarried. The choice of a celibate way of life in a vowed religious context differs somewhat from the celibacy which is chosen, perhaps temporarily, for a variety of reasons. Some may be self-transcendent, others ego-centric, or some again occurring through the circumstances of life. Viewed from a Christian standpoint, celibacy, no matter the reason for its choice, presupposes ideally an abstention from genital activity. It is in this sense that I shall use the term, celibate, even while recognising that many single people in today's world are sexually active. As marriage most commonly provides the context for the adult to develop affectively and grow in intimacy with a spouse and children, the celibate must face the challenge of developing affectivity and growing to intimacy and generativity outside this usual setting.

The need to cultivate the affective dimension applies especially to those who have chosen a vowed celibate way of life that they may be more readily available to serve others. Compassion, empathy, and the gift of self, all find their source in this area of our being. The aim of this dimension of sexuality is to reach out to others, to touch them deeply and allow ourselves to be touched in return. This is what is meant by intimacy. To be intimate with another is not something which can be effected at will; it comes as a gift, enriching life, but it can also be a difficult and demanding process, filled as it is with exigencies. Erikson speaks of intimacy as 'the capacity to commit oneself to concrete affiliations and partnerships and to develop the ethical strength to abide by such commitments, even though they call for significant sacrifices and compromises'.[3] Such closeness can be a continuing source of wonder and mystery. It can be an end in itself or may be a prelude to and accompaniment of genital intimacy.

For the celibate it is important to be aware of what is being sought in intimacy. Is the object close friendship or is it seeking a genital relationship with another? This is a question which must be faced openly by any who do not wish for a relationship to become genital. Because affective and genital sexuality are so closely linked, it is not unusual that intimacy with another on the affective level will result in some tie-in of genitality. This may be the case particularly during mid-life when genital needs can reach a new ascendancy. There is no need to be overly concerned about such stirrings or desires as long as the celibate remains in a position to control them. If the aim is to keep the relationship on an affective level and genital behaviour can be controlled, even though there may be quite a normal desire for this, then the friendship remains a healthy celibate one. A mature adult knows for the most part when his or her way of acting is demonstrating affection and when it is giving rise to or encouraging a genital response.

Heterosexual friendships, as well as those with members of one's own sex, are a significant means of developing both sides of the personality. It is through such companionship that we come to know ourselves as woman or man and to bring into consciousness much of the opposite-sexed attributes of the personality. Again, if these relationships are to remain celibate, it is important to be aware that men and women react differently. Touch, a valuable and beautiful avenue of affection, can in many cases, especially in men, be highly stimulating genitally. Experience enables a person to know how best to communicate feeling in the way desired. Women religious have often been amazed and shocked when a man has made genital advances to them, after they have acted in a way which for them was simply engaging, while for the man was highly seductive.

Such heterosexual relationships may not be easy to keep from becoming genital. It requires a considerable amount of strength to do so and this is best achieved through self-discipline and prayer.

Intimacy and friendship are vital also for psychological health. Absence of the possibility of sharing aspirations, desires or difficulties at the level of self-revelation has been found to correlate positively with certain psychosomatic illnesses. Those who cannot risk the challenges and wonder of meeting and sharing with another at depth become tense, repressed and brittle in their relationships. They face the inevitable results of stress in their bodies and psyches.

There is a need in all of us to open ourselves at depth to another, to be known and to be loved. The challenge of intimacy is to be able to meet this need appropriately in a reciprocal relationship without becoming possessive in our loving, too demanding or exclusive. Once we have encountered another in this way, and experienced our own loveableness we are more readily open to accept God's love into the core of our being and to recognise the yearning of the human spirit for communion with him.

Genital sexuality

The final dimension of sexuality that we need to look at is the genital. For many, this has been equated with the whole area of sexuality, but to disregard the other equally important aspects is to be too narrow in our understanding. The genital drive is sometimes spoken of as consisting of two facets: genitality and genital behaviour. Genitality refers to the erotic desires, thoughts, stirrings, feelings of stimulation and fantasies which may or may not lead to genital behaviour. Such behaviour or activity is that which is designed to culminate in orgasm.

To reach maturity means not only a psychological, spiritual and intellectual maturity. It means also full sexual maturity, including the genital dimension. This does not necessarily imply genital activity, but it does require a full possession of oneself as a sexual being. It is, perhaps, the area of genital sexuality which is the least well integrated in most people, whether sexually active or not. There are many reasons for this, some the result of faulty development, others of defence mechanisms such as denial or repression.

In describing psychosexual growth and development Michael Cavanagh speaks of three major stages: childhood, adolescence and adulthood.[4] Within each stage he recognises steps or phases — three in the first two stages, with two phases in adulthood. Healthy development supposes a normal passage from one phase to the next. However, this progress may be slowed by internal or external factors so that psychosexual growth is stunted. Or again the person may fixate at one level and fail to develop further. As in all development, stages cannot be skipped and failure to negotiate one stage must be recognised and remedied before the next can proceed.

In the first two years of childhood, the time of Sexual Unawareness, sexual identity is weak and finds its source in the way the child is treated, whether as boy or girl. Although children may play with their genitals and apparently reach orgasm, the experience differs from that of the adult. If parents react too strongly to this in a way which threatens the child, he or she may fixate at this level for an indefinite period. Adults who have thus fixated in childhood and have never developed beyond this first phase are asexual, experiencing no genital pleasure or interest even within marriage, or other loving sexual relationship.

The second phase of childhood sexuality is that of Sexual Awakening, between the ages of three and seven. The discovery in the little girl or little boy of the difference in their bodies leads to a degree of excitement and curiosity, often accompanied by sex-play with others. There may be an increase in masturbation especially if the child has little other engaging occupation. Should the child fixate at this level through lack of satisfying occupation and diversion, genital activity in adulthood will be experienced as threatening and embarrassing. There may also be an inclination to turn to children or members of the same sex for genital satisfaction. This is an age at which children are particularly sensitive to the reaction of their elders. Parents who can calmly and firmly instruct their children to distinguish between acceptable and non-acceptable ways of acting without being over-harsh or threatening, will help them move to the subsequent developmental phase of Sexual Surreptitiousness.

This is the time between the ages of approximately seven and twelve when there is an apparent loss of interest in the genital. In actuality this is not the case. Children appear to have learnt that the area of sexuality is something best concealed from their parents and, while sex-play and interest in sexual material is growing, they are careful to keep it hidden. Their secretiveness about sexual activity or desire will persist into adulthood if fixation takes place at this stage.

Healthy development readies the child for the approach of adolescence. During the span of the teen years, attitudes — whether positive or negative — learned in childhood will be either reinforced or, in some cases, modified. The phase of Sexual Fantasy with self or with others enables adolescents to integrate 'the intellect and emotions with genital sexuality' and to move gradually to a more other-centred sexuality, rehearsing, as it were, sexual behaviours in their minds. Lack of social opportunity or fear of heterosexual relationships may lead to fixation at this point. Adults who have fixated at this phase will tend to restrict their sexual lives to fantasy or at least find more satisfaction there than in a physical relationship.

As the body matures and develops, genital interest tends to absorb the middle adolescent, and the phase of Sexual Preoccupation commences. Masturbation is frequent, especially amongst boys, and while the girls become 'boy mad', their counterparts are marking up their 'conquests'. This 'sexual saturation' eventually allows the young person to settle down and reach a sense of balance. Failure, through shyness or lack of opportunity, to move out into some type of heterosexual relationship can result in fixation. If this is not worked through, the adult will remain preoccupied with sex in subsequent years to the detriment of other interests and values.

The final phase in adolescence Cavanagh refers to as Superficial Sexual Relating. This is a time of experimenting in relationships and finding one's way with members of the opposite sex. Socialising in groups and dating play an important part in discovering one's sexual identity. The relationship is still very self-centred as well as self-conscious. It is possible to fixate at this stage through fear of moving to a closer intimacy, sometimes because of insecurity or lack of self-confidence. Such a person will not be able to enter a deeper relationship and will remain narcissistic in his or her dealings with others.

Adult Sexuality, the third stage of sexual development, commences with the phase of 'Psychosexual Mutuality'. The young adult progresses from the self-centredness of the preceding stage to a desire to meet another with respect, love and tenderness. The twenties are usually the years of greatest genital need in the man, sometimes spoken of as sexual peaking, whereas this may not be experienced by the woman until her thirties or forties.

Full sexual maturity is reached usually by about thirty years of age and continues throughout the second half of life. Cavanagh gives the name Psychosexual Integration to this phase which is a time when genital needs find their balance among other equally important values and interests.

Genital desire may wane in the later years of life but this is not necessarily the case. Many find their needs increase rather than diminish. Erikson tells of one ninety-two-year-old man whose wife was obliged to sleep in a downstairs bedroom to care for her invalided sister. His one complaint about this arrangement was: 'It's ruined my sex life, but I don't think she did this on purpose.'[5]

Genital sexuality is a part of our totality that is frequently not integrated into the rest of living. This is not only the case with celibates but is found also among sexually active single people and not infrequently in marriage. The main reason for this seems to be a failure in education and fear or disgust rather than a wonder at the beauty of this power that we hold, whether or not we choose to exercise it.

Many people have repressed their genitality, blocking the awareness of genital impulses and successfully keeping any interest or desire in this area out of consciousness. This is a defence mechanism used to ward off anxiety, guilt or fear, and often results from parental attitudes in early life or sometimes from some sexual trauma, especially in the case of women. To repress any emotion or need requires a degree of energy which can be draining. It is at mid-life, especially, that all areas of repression require more and more energy to hold them out of consciousness. This invariably leads to frustration, irritability and often anger. As is the case with all repressed material, there is a tendency to project on to the other what we refuse to accept ourselves. So it is that such a person, for example a member of a religious community, will begin to see in other members of the community an obsession with sexual matters. This can be the cause of becoming inordinately judgemental and righteous in one's own views.

But we cannot normally repress indefinitely. Finally there will come an explosion of sexuality. What happens in this case is that a regression takes place back to the stage of sexual development at which the repression first occurred. Sexual needs at that level become exaggerated. It is necessry then to work through this and the following steps before full maturity is reached. A woman of forty-five was amazed to find herself highly excited both genitally and socially after moving into a friendship with the local pastor. 'It seemed,' she said, 'as though I was acting like an adolescent', and this was precisely what was happening. She had successfully blocked awareness of any genital needs since puberty and now, with a sudden release of the repression, found herself acting out in an adolescent fashion. Fortunately, it does not take as much time in later life to work through the various levels as it does during normal development.

Cavanagh points out that when a regression of this type takes place, it is important to understand that the criteria used to judge any morality involved must be those of the appropriate age for that particular stage, rather than those applied to adult behaviour. Moral criteria for the young child or adolescent differ from the standards applied to the adult and this must be taken into consideration in making moral judgements. 'Childhood and adolescence are psychological stages far more than they are chronological ranges. A thirty-year-old man or a fifty-year-old woman, through no fault of his or her own, may be going through delayed psychosexual development, which may take years to complete. Although these people are chronologically adults, their sexual behaviour is still developmental and should be judged accordingly.'[6]

While a repression lasts, we are never really free from the emotions or desires repressed, even though unaware of their existence. Not only do they influence our behaviour in spite of our unawareness but finally in some way they will take possession of us. Repression then is an unhealthy and destructive way of handling sexuality.

Suppression, also a defence mechanism, is very different. Genital feelings and longings are acknowledged but we decide, for some good reason, to put them aside and give our attention to other occupations. This is not always easy to achieve and requires considerable self-control.

Sublimation implies directing the energy which might otherwise express itself genitally, into some other acceptable activity. This is a means used often by adolescents and young adults who have chosen a celibate way of life. A hard game of some sport or an energetic tramp through the countryside can help the young person keep control over his or her sexual needs.

Suppression and sublimation have their place in the sexual life. They can be healthy and helpful. However, they do not help to integrate this area of genitality, making it a recognised and welcome part of our integral personhood.

How then can we develop and fully integrate genitality in a way that is healthy and appropriate to our position in life? To do this implies coming to value this aspect of our personhood through which we can express ourselves intimately with another, and in which can be found one of the highest human pleasures. This does not necessitate genital behaviour or activity, but it does presuppose an appreciation of and a respect for this power, even when for good reasons the choice is made not to exercise it. Many celibate people have reached a higher degree of self-actualisation in this area than have some genitally active couples. To integrate genital sexuality means to acknowledge that the genital dimension is part of the whole person. It is one of the ways in which we can come to a knowledge of ourselves as integral people, vital and loving, and reveal this to another.

Such an expression of the whole human person is a revelation, an articulation, of a rational spiritual being, consisting not only of body but also of mind and of spirit. Erotic sensations and impulses are not simply reflexes centred in the genital organs. Because we are human, rather than purely animal, the true centre of genital sexuality is in the brain. Our sexual energies, just as all our human energies, must be regulated rationally, must find their direction in the reflective mind. Thus we are enabled to respond to another thoughtfully and with care rather than merely reacting erotically. Because we are human rather than animal our genital relations can tell of love and of commitment; can be non-possessive, tender and caring.

To integrate sexuality means not simply to use these powers functionally, unrelated to the rest of our being, or to look on another purely as a sex partner without reference to the rest of his or her personhood. It means rather to be fully aware of genital stirrings, desires or urges and to let them find their true centre; to allow the energy created genitally to be directed to the mind; to live a reflective sexual life. It means to learn to express these impulses, or to refrain from doing so, in a way that does not strive to possess the other in eroticism, but aims to respect the whole of his or her being while understanding and reverencing our own.

To direct these impulses to their inner centre is to give full expression to them, an acceptance not a repression, and an opportunity for amplification as they reach new depths in awareness, appreciation and understanding. This will enrich a subsequent outward expression in genital activity with an integral person rather than a purely genital sex-mate. One then becomes aware of the totality of sexuality knowing oneself to be a warm, affectionate and caring man or woman in an intimate union with another person whose whole being is reverenced and respected.

To experience sexual feelings or longings, then, gives an opportunity to recognise ourselves as individuals gifted with the power of procreating the human race, as well as of moving to the closest possible manifestation of intimacy with another. If we accept the presence of these stirrings and see in them an utterance or revelation of the person we really are, we come to appreciate ourselves as fully woman or man. We know ourselves capable of self-giving and of receiving another in love, whether or not we intend to enjoy this possibility. Not only does such an approach move us to a fresh awareness of self but with that awareness comes a new respect and esteem for others.

For just as the appraisal of any reality depends on the attitude held towards it, so will the understanding of genital sexuality be experienced according to the stance taken towards it. Those who look no further than the erotic, will register only that. For those who can see deeper, a whole world of wonder at the beauty of oneself and another can be savoured. We see and experience what we are prepared to perceive. Just as an artist who happens upon a forest of trees might be aware of the harmony of light and shade, of colour and form, of the rhythm of branches and trunks; a botanist be struck by the species of trees, of ferns and of flowers; a carpenter by the texture of each variety of wood; so, too, we see what our eyes have been trained to appreciate. A masterpiece depicting the nude body will be for some a revelation of the beauty of the human form, an expresson of true manhood or womanhood. For others, it may be the equivalent of erotica. They become fixated and aroused at the genital level, unable to see beyond the breasts of a woman, the penis of a man; unable to move to an appreciation of the person possessing these sexual organs, to value the aesthetic.

It is this ability to move to the deepest reality which is being revealed that enables us to freely integrate the spontaneous genital feelings, desires and fantasies. 'Reveal' comes from the Latin root, *re* meaning un — and *velare* veil. It is when we can look again and see the true personhood of another, and of ourselves, revealed or 'unveiled' through this genital articulation that we learn to respect the dignity and beauty of genital sexuality which is one way of giving expression to our human integrity.

Genital sexuality then is just as much a part of integral personhood as is affective sexuality and it is one way in which the whole person is revealed at depth. Genital relationships are a means of manifesting who we truly are, hopefully loving, integrated individuals who are ready to give of ourselves, and are drawn to share deeply with another. Such a meeting gives expression to the whole personality. The central motivating force of this relationship should be love, but it is important to understand that the genital behaviour is not in itself the love. 'Love is a deeper thing. We enter into its deepest reality,' Raguin tells us, 'by disassociating it from the signs that manifest it.'[7] Men sometimes confuse love with genitality, while women often confuse it with emotional satisfaction and reassurance. In these cases the depth of love is never experienced and its profoundest reality never fathomed.

Genital desire or behaviour is not always motivated by genital need but may arise from a variety of causes. Loneliness, a poor self-image, tension at work, anxiety and stress can all show themselves as an apparent need for genital behaviour, especially in the form of masturbation. These cravings are, however, not based in sexuality at all. The longing to be affirmed and accepted as man or as woman may also give rise to intense genital stirrings. Affective needs such as the yearning to be touched, held, hugged or to be really cared for by another are not infrequently linked with genital desire. A dream relating to intercourse showed one young woman that what she was seeking in reality was not a genital relationship, but rather to be held closely by someone who loved her, in order to compensate for the lack of expressed affection in her earlier years. As well, hormonal changes or the emergences into consciousness of the anima or animus, and the need to integrate this contrasexual side of the personality, are often exposed through some type of genital desire or fantasy.

It is important to see what all such impulses, desires or fantasies are bringing to light. It is their cause that attention needs to be focused on rather than the manifestation. This will facilitate a constructive handling of the situation which is developmental and enriching instead of being immature or destructive.

There is a close connection between sexuality, in each of its three dimensions, and spirituality. True freedom in the area of sexuality is reflected in the ability to relate with ease, warmth and maturity to others. It is also linked with our highest spiritual aspirations. Gerald May maintains that the sexual drive and the longing for union with God have 'a common root force'.[8] Stunting in the one area invariably leads to a certain crippling in the other and our relationship with God lacks freedom and spontaneity. Fear of genital energy and drive is accompanied by a fear of closeness to God. A mature and integrated sexuality can lead unerringly to a deep spiritual communion and an ability to experience something of the mystery of divine love.

Sexuality in the consecrated celibate at mid-life

For many vowed celibates the middle years can be a time of becoming acutely aware of genital needs which have not previously entered consciousness. While for the majority this can be an enriching and integrating experience, for others it becomes a disturbing and confusing embarrassment. Failure to understand the reason for this unexpected revelation of womanhood or manhood can lead to a belief that celibate life is no longer a possibility. Indeed, many have left religious life, or have moved into a de facto relationship, only to discover that this was no real solution to their difficulties and failed to bring the fulfilment that they sought.

Deepening needs for intimacy at this time of life may well lead into relationships which tend to stimulate previously repressed or undeveloped genital needs. It can happen that the time of Sexual Preoccupation or Superficial Sexual Relating has been delayed through lack of opportunity to meet with members of the opposite sex, or excessive occupation in earlier years. Involvement in a heavy programme of study at this age has often a similar effect. Sexual peaking will then also be delayed.

For many, mid-life is the time when repressed sexuality explodes leaving them confused and bewildered by the strength and urgency of genital desire which has not been experienced before. The woman or man in the late thirties, the forties or fifties may be faced with urgent genital needs which become increasingly difficult to control. This can be complicated by the possibility that an infatuation, similar to that encountered in adolescence, may occur at this stage of life. The overwhelming attraction towards another can become so powerful that nothing short of a genital response can appear sufficient to satisfy the need to give of oneself and to meet the one loved at the depth desired.

Loneliness, a frequent accompaniment of the time of crisis, may be a further complicating factor. This together with the need to be affirmed in one's masculinity or femininity may pressure the celibate into a relationship which inclines towards genital expression and a questioning of the commitment to celibacy.

For the celibate who is faced with these overpowering genital desires and who does not understand what is happening, there can appear to be no escape apart from leaving the present life-style and seeking satisfaction of these needs in marriage. For the woman, who may well be experiencing the normal longing for motherhood, the urgency to move into a new way of life is great as the possibility of bearing a child is lessening with each passing year.

It is no wonder then that so many in religious life face a crisis in commitment during the years of mid-life. Not only may they be confronted with a struggle in the area of sexuality but like others their questioning extends to ministry, to faith and to their very relationship with God. They, too, can become filled with ennui, listless and trapped as they face the classroom, the hospital ward or the parish office each morning. They, too, can see the grass greener on the other side of the fence.

For any decision to be balanced and honest a certain peace of mind is necessary to see and weigh options clearly. To try to decide about a future course of action, while factors such as those mentioned above are still in a state of turbulence, can lead to a wrong choice of alternatives. For a wise and considered decision, time must be allowed for the situation to settle, for emotions to calm and for circumstances to fall into place. Only then can we see where we are truly called. The midst of crisis is never the best time for prudent decision making. A crisis of this kind may well be the prelude to a deeper and richer living out of the celibate way of life, one in which weakness, and perhaps sinfulness, is acknowledged and true love and compassion learned.

Many celibate people do not undergo this type of experience at mid-life and find that these years are relatively uneventful as far as their genitality is concerned. But for all, the middle years should provide a time of fathoming and enriching their appreciation of being a fully sexual man or woman.

Marriage and mid-life

Profound changes are taking place in both the man

and the woman during their middle years and this has its repercussions in their marriage. We have seen that the norm is for the woman to face the mid-life transition several years younger than the man, but it is also common for women to marry men some years their senior. Such a situation results in both meeting the crisis at approximately the same time. In other instances one partner may be passing through a time of turbulence and trauma about which the other knows nothing.

The boredom, emptiness, dissatisfaction and depression accompanying these years all have their ramifications in the marriage. 'Year after year, after year the same face is there to greet you at the breakfast table, to lie on the pillow beside you each night,' complained one forty-year-old. Unless new meaning is found in the marriage as both partners change and as children leave the home, there can be little hope that the union will deepen and be enriched, or even remain intact. This cannot be achieved without some mutual sharing and openness, a readiness to discuss what is happening to each other, the changing needs each is experiencing, their interests and aspirations. This can prove difficult for those who have never really talked to one another in the earlier years of marriage, who have never reached an intimacy that allows for true communication. Such exchange leads to a mutual respect of the tensions and problems each is facing — the added pressures at work and feelings of inadequacy for the man; and perhaps for the woman, even one who has worked outside the house, the loneliness and growing sense of resentment and anger that her life has been so restricted by the needs of husband and children.

Changes in sexuality must be recognised and understood. The woman needs to appreciate the effect on her husband of the gradual fall-off in the production of the male hormone, testosterone. There can be a resultant decline in sexual responsiveness: arousal takes longer and it becomes more difficult to maintain an erection. For those who have tended to identify their masculinity with sexual potency this is perceived as a threat to their self-esteem. An added complication may well be that the wife is becoming more sophisticated and assertive in her sexual needs which can be reaching their highest point at the time when her husband's potency is beginning to wane. This can constitute a real threat to the man who is perhaps becoming uncertain as to his ability to perform sexually.

Many an affair with a younger and less experienced partner starts as a consequence. The older man may be flattered by the response of a young and attractive woman which proves stimulating, not only genitally, but also to his self-esteem.

We have seen also how a man can well project the seductive and alluring aspect of his anima onto a woman outside the home and in consequence be strongly attracted by her. This can be accompanied by a previous projection of the less attractive aspect, which usually surfaces first, onto the closest woman to him, namely his wife. It is not difficult then to foresee the results. If, however, the wife understands what is happening and does not allow herself to live out his projection of the irritable, negative woman; if she does not permit her aggressive animus to hit back, but rather can remain silent and wait, her husband will be free to re-own his projection and find his balance and direction once more.

As the woman's need for intimacy is deepening more rapidly than the man's at this stage of life, it becomes even more pressing for her to *feel* that she is loved and appreciated. So often this is taken for granted by the man in marriage. Surely the fact that his life is spent in providing and caring for his wife is sufficient evidence of his affection. But the woman has a deep need for repeated re-assurance. How often a mid-life woman has said to me: 'If only he would tell me that he loves me, or just put his arms around me at times.'

As business concerns become more critical, there is often little time or energy left for mid-life men to cultivate their sexual lives. For them 'quick sex' can be satisfying and sufficient. For women this is rarely so and can be disappointing and destructive to the relationship. What they look for in a genital relationship is the re-assurance that they are loved and valued.

Neither has the woman the same ability or desire to compartmentalise her life as has a man. For her a disagreement earlier in the day must be worked through and forgiven before she can enjoy a genital relationship at night. Intercourse for her is not an isolated act as it may be for her husband, but is in continuity with the rest of living.

When the years around menopause approach, an informed and understanding husband can ease many of the difficulties which may face his wife. We shall look later at these in more depth. Suffice it to say in the words of one man: 'We men should make it our business to give our wives the support they need during the time of menopause. As it is, we know little about it and do even less.'

As both the woman and man find deep personality changes occurring with the emergence of their authentic self, a re-working of identity takes place. Whenever the sense of identity falters there invariably follows a loss in the ability to sustain intimacy. This, combined with the general emotional volatility at mid-life, can lead to an overwhelming infatuation followed by a period of alienation. This falling in love and falling out of love can be the source of many affairs on the part of both partners. But it is said that such an association, if based purely on infatuation, will have a life span of little more than six months.

These complex changes necessitate a re-appraisal of the meaning of the marriage which alters as the partners mature and children leave the home. The challenge is there to move to a more profound level of intimacy and acceptance of changing needs and more flexible roles. For the married couple who have successfully integrated their sexuality, the second half of life can offer a far richer sexual relationship in which love and intimacy reach a degree of union unattainable in earlier life.

♦ ♦ ♦

Chapter • 9

MENOPAUSE AND THE CLIMACTERIC

There is confusion in the minds of many about the various changes which confront both women and men during their years of mid-life. Arguments persist as to whether or not there is such a phenomenon as a 'male menopause' or whether it is solely a female experience. A tissue of myths still shrouds the truth about menopause and these myths have, in the past, given rise to a real fear of this normal physiological transition.

Fortunately now women are, for the most part, approaching this time in their lives with a more balanced and prosaic attitude, some even with a sense of relief and anticipation of a life free from many of the anxieties which have been theirs. As one put it: 'I can't wait to have the hassles of menstruation or an unwanted pregnancy behind me, and to be able to enjoy life to the full.' For her there were none of the worries about losing her femininity or attractiveness which weigh on some women. She was looking forward to a life just as full as she had always known, aware that she could maintain her sexual attraction and capacity.

Women approach this time of life with a variety of feelings as Bernice Neugarten[1] discovered when she researched the attitudes to menopause of women of different ages. The middle-aged group, on the whole, regarded the change as less significant than did the younger, and seemed more confident of being able to cope with any difficulties. Acknowledging that it was 'an unpleasant time and perhaps a little frightening', most were able to look forward to a time in the postmenopausal period when they would be 'both happier and healthier'. Postmenopausal zest, PMZ, is now becoming far more widely acclaimed.

In order to clarify the changes that are occurring at this stage of life it is necessary to distinguish between three distinct phenomena which are frequently confused and misunderstood: the mid-life transition or crisis, the climacteric and menopause.

The transition, as we have seen, is a time of possible upheaval and turmoil in almost every area of life, affecting both men and women between the ages of approximately thirty-five and forty-five. Underlying this, but distinct from it, may be the climacteric. In many instances, especially in the case of men, this does not, however, start until later. The climacteric refers to the gradual loss of the reproductive ability in both sexes as a result of a decrease in the production of the sex hormones specific to each. Finally, menopause is the technical term given to the cessation of menstruation, and is, therefore, specific to women. There is no such entity as a 'male menopause', though there is a 'male climacteric', despite how many might like to deny it.

To comprehend these very complex changes requires some understanding of the endocrine system in the body. Hormones, which stimulate the activity of many bodily organs, are secreted from a series of ductless endocrine glands and are liberated directly into the bloodstream to be carried to the parts of the body under their control. Most people are far more acquainted with the action of a hormone like thyroxin from the thyroid gland than they are with that of the sex hormones: oestrogen and progesterone which predominate in the woman, and testosterone in the man. Oestrogen is responsible for the development and maintenance of female traits in the woman, while testosterone is related to the masculine characteristics of the man. These hormones are produced for the most part by the ovaries or the testes, a lesser amount of both being manufactured also by the adrenal glands. Both types of hormones are, therefore, present in each sex, though that secreted by the adrenals plays little part in reproduction.

The production of the sex hormones, as of all hormones, is under the control of the pituitary gland which lies carefully protected in a small cavity in the lower part of the skull. The pituitary has been called by some 'the conductor of the orchestra' as it is responsible for the harmonious functioning of many areas of the body. It, in its turn, is controlled in this role by the hypothalamus at the base of the brain. If we were to explore further, it would become evident that the hypothalamus forms a bridge, as it were, with the exterior world and is influenced by changes wrought in our mental and emotional states by factors both internal and external. This explains the disturbance to the menstrual cycle resulting from shock, stress or even a change of country.

The pituitary gland produces two gonadotropins, which are the same in both male and female: follicle-stimulating hormone, known as FSH; and luteinizing hormone, LH, which is sometimes called interstitial-cell-stimulating hormone, ICSH, in the male. These two are responsible for stimulating the production of the sex hormones in the adrenals and the specific sex glands or gonads. In the woman this takes place in a cyclic pattern, while in the man it is more constant and non-cyclic.

The very complex female cycle may be simply described as a process whereby a certain number of egg-containing follicles in the ovaries are stimulated each month by FSH to mature and produce oestrogen. The oestrogen has an effect on the sense of well-being, the moods and many other areas of the woman's life. It also begins the preparation for a possible pregnancy by commencing the build-up of the endometrial lining of the womb or uterus. At about twelve days from the commencement of the cycle, one, or possibly more, ova or eggs are liberated into the fallopian tube from a rupture of one or more follicles. Occasionally there may be no egg within the follicle and an anovulatory cycle occurs with no chance of a pregnancy. This is common in early adolescence and towards the end of the woman's reproductive life. This part of the cycle is controlled by LH from the pituitary gland. The follicle continues to secrete oestrogen and now also progesterone which completes the preparation of the endometrium for the implantation of a possible pregnancy. If the ovum remains unfertilised, chemical messages reach the pituitary which in turn signals the follicle, now known as the corpus luteum, to cease the production of hormones. As the blood level of oestrogen and progesterone drops, the thickened endometrium is shed in the menstrual period and another cycle commences under the influence of FSH. Should the ovum be fertilised the corpus luteum continues its secretion of hormone thus maintaining the pregnancy and preventing the production of FSH by the pituitary. The cyclic pattern of hormone production is broken and recurs only after the pregnancy ends.

In the case of the man, the secretion of FSH and ICSH from the pituitary is constant and is regulated by the level of testosterone in the blood. The FSH stimulates the sperm formation in the testes while the ICSH is responsible for controlling the secretion of testosterone by the interstitial cells. The role of testosterone is one that affects the whole male body. It not only determines masculine development and traits but it influences sexual desire and libido, and also acts upon other body systems such as the central nervous system, the vascular system and the balance between tissue fluids and salts. Like oestrogen it affects emotional well-being, energy level and the ability to withstand stress.

As both the ovaries and testes age they become no longer able to respond to the stimulation of FSH and LH in the same way. Less and less of the sex hormones are secreted over the years of the climacteric. Ovulation gradually declines and ceases, as does also the production of sperm. By the age of forty most women have probably begun to experience some drop in the hormone level, though others may vary considerably in this. This change seems to occur later in men, usually in the late forties to the sixties, though this again differs from one individual to another. Some have been known to father children into their eighties and even nineties.

The gradual transition from the reproductive to the non-reproductive era is completed only when the body reaches a new and different state of hormonal balance. It is spread over a widely varying number of years, usually longer in the man than in the woman. This time of the climacteric is referred to by some as the 'change of life'.

Menopause

Menopause occurs at the point in the climacteric when the fall in oestrogen production is such that it no longer builds up the endometrium sufficiently for a menstrual period to take place. Because of the usual irregularities in menstruation at this stage, the exact moment of menopause may be difficult to ascertain. Periods may be missed during the two to three years before menopause and some women report having stopped menstruating for several months or even up to a year and then recommencing their menstrual periods. It is usually recognised that menopause has occurred if there has been no period for over a year. Not only can there be an irregularity in the periods before menopause for most women but this may be accompanied by a very scant or occasionally very heavy flow. As these years are also a time when uterine cancer is common in women any untoward bleeding during or between periods or after intercourse should be reported and checked medically.

Though the time of menopause varies widely, some women reaching it by forty or earlier, the average age would appear to be between forty-five and fifty-five. There does not seem to be any link at all between the time of the menarche (onset of the periods) in adolescence and that of the menopause in mid-life. There does, however, appear to be some heredity influence, early or late menopause being a common feature in certain families. Research at Boston University School of Medicine has also demonstrated clearly that smoking results in an early menopause. This may be due to the effects of nicotine on hormone secretions, but the cause is still not clear.

About twenty per cent of women suffer no adverse symptoms during the years surrounding menopause. This is probably due to a very gradual change in oestrogen production. A more sudden drop, for instance that resulting from surgical removal of the ovaries, is frequently associated with more severe symptoms. Most women are affected in ways that vary from being mildly inconveniencing to 'bothersome but manageable'. About fifteen per cent, however, may become sufficiently distressed as to require medical help and counselling.

What is it that gives rise to such a variety of complaints? As less and less oestrogen is produced, the pituitary gland in an all-out effort to stimulate the ovaries, pours out more and more FSH leading to turmoil in the hormonal balance. This, in turn, affects the hypothalamus which is responsible not only for the normal functioning of the pituitary, but for a variety of bodily functions. Among these are heat control, sleep, energy levels and the autonomic nervous system which controls among other things, the contraction and dilatation of blood vessels and the activity of the sweat glands. Malfunctioning of the hypothalamus from a low oestrogen level can, therefore, give rise to all manner of symptoms in every part of the body.

The most common among these are hot flushes or flashes which may or may not be accompanied by perspiration. These result from the instability of the vasomotor system or blood vessels. It is not uncommon for this type of disturbance to start the year or so prior to menopause and to continue for some years after it. Flushes may occur on the odd occasion and be fairly mild, or they may come as an experience of intense heat and flushing, usually from the waist up, ten to twelve times a day. They may last for a few seconds or for up to fifteen minutes or more. Mild perspiration or profuse sweating can accompany the experience which is particularly prone to occur at night. Some women have had to change their sheets several times in the one night. This can lead to very troubled sleep not only for the woman concerned but also for her partner.

Fortunately, this is one of the most easily controlled of the menopausal symptoms. Flushes occurring during the day may not be obvious in any way to others, unless the sufferer announces in the middle of winter that it is becoming very warm and then proceeds to open all the windows! This will bring an out-cry from others who are not similarly affected at that particular moment.

Other symptoms like tingling, numbness or crawling sensations, cramps, insomnia, faintness or dizzy spells, lack of energy, palpitations, emotional disturbances and headaches may all be associated with the fluctuating hormonal level. Often irritability, weepiness and tiredness are also secondary results of sleepless nights or anxiety caused by some of the above happenings.

Many of the so-called menopausal symptoms, depression for example, have little to do with menopause, but are caused by other events occurring at this time. Some women approach the normal ageing process as the end of usefulness or attractiveness and this in itself can be depressing. A husband too pre-occupied with business affairs to give his wife the attention she craves can create self-doubt. Again, many are facing a death in the family for the first time at mid-life. Research seems to indicate that there is no such thing as menopausal depression, though depression may well occur around these years for other reasons.

Occasionally, women will act 'out of character' at this time of life, shoplifting or defiantly breaking traffic regulations. The exact cause of this is unknown but it may well be a cry for attention or help during these years which are more critical for some than for others.

The ovaries continue to secrete a gradually lessening amount of hormone after menopause takes place and will keep doing so for a number of years. As oestrogen balance appears to play a part in the absorption of calcium, women, and to a lesser extent men, are likely to develop oesteoporosis during this part of the climacteric unless additional calcium is supplied. Osteoporosis reveals itself in brittleness of bones resulting in repeated fractures, and in the rounded and humped back from changes in the vertebrae with a consequent loss of height.

The mucous membranes of the body are also affected as the level of oestrogen drops in the postmenopausal period. Dryness and thinning of the vaginal wall may cause difficulties in intercourse and this can be relieved by the use of a cream. Drier nasal membranes and a lessened flow of saliva may at times give rise to alterations in smell and taste.

Other postmenopausal changes which occur only after ten or fifteen years are a shrinkage of the vulva and vagina, as well as of the uterus and ovaries. Hair thins in various areas of the body, including the pubic area, while at the same time the growth of facial hair, which commenced much earlier, may thicken and darken.

This sounds a sad litany of complaints, certainly

sufficient to cause some trepidation in the hearts of most. But the majority of women experience only a few symptoms and in a way that causes little inconvenience.

For those unable to cope with their menopausal symptoms hormonal replacement therapy, HRT, can be effective in bringing some relief. Hot flushes, sweating and vaginal dryness all respond positively to supplementary oestrogen which brings with it also a restoration of the sense of well-being and renewed energy. Whether or not other symptoms are eased will depend on whether they are actually caused by the sex hormone deficiency in the first place.

The more usual HRT now involves not only a replacement of the oestrogen but also of the progesterone, and will result in a slight menstrual-like bleeding. The addition of a progestogen, the synthetic form of progesterone, to the therapy lessens the danger of endometrial cancer, making it a far safer option for all, except those suffering from breast cancer, liver disease or thromboembolic disorders. Contrary to the belief of many women, this therapy does not delay or prolong the menopausal process as the body responds to its own rhythm and will in time recover its balance.

Those unable or unwilling to use HRT may find that clonidine will ease the hot flushing though this is not successful in all cases. Other suggested remedies range through vitamins to health foods but there is little proof of their efficacy. However, if anything is found to be helpful it is worth using, as long as it is not detrimental to health in other ways. An oestrogen cream can ease the drying and possible irritation of the vagina, but the oestrogen will be absorbed into the bloodstream and may, therefore, be inadvisable in the cases mentioned above.

The male climacteric

The climacteric in men brings with it consequences which in many ways parallel some of those experienced by women. Since testosterone has such a wide-ranging effect on the body tissues, emotional stability and well-being, its diminution is reflected in these areas. The pituitary gland reacts to the falling level of testosterone by an increased production of FSH and ICSH resulting in an imbalance of hormones. This then affects the hypothalamus giving rise to disturbances such as loss of energy, sleep disorders, emotional instability, metabolic changes, lessened libido and sometimes impotence. Finally the production of sperm ceases bringing to an end the possibility of reproduction. The whole process extends over a longer period in men and probably for this reason the symptoms are not as obvious as they are in women.

Memory loss

Memory loss, whether or not influenced at all by the hormonal level, can be a further hazard of the middle years. How often we stand before an open cupboard wondering why on earth we are there. What was it that made us open it in the first place? Decline in short-term memory may start around the mid-forties or earlier, and it becomes evident in countless ways. Names of friends, no matter how long we have known them, tend to escape our minds just as we make an introduction, only to pop back unexpectedly a few minutes later — unfortunately too late. It can be hard to recall immediately what day of the week it is, for some even what year they are in. Memory blanks are common and the tip-of-the-tongue phenomenon, when that needed word escapes us, makes speaking in public hazardous. It is little wonder, then, that many people fear that they may be losing their sanity.

The loss is not one of intelligence but rather of speed of recall, which may in fact improve again later. It can be helped greatly by making associations which create links in the brain leading to the lost name, word or article. Younger people tend to do this automatically. With age our memory bank becomes more crowded and we often become 'untidy' or disorderly in the storage of information making it difficult to find what we are seeking amidst the clutter. Memory aids or mnemonics can help to re-establish order and train us to the level of concentration and discipline necessary to retrieve stored information. Someone used significant dates in her life to remember a telephone number when needed. Recall, however, will probably never again be as sharp as it was at age sixteen.

♦ ♦ ♦

Chapter • 10

TOWARDS A SPIRITUALITY OF MID-LIFE

The movement into and through the middle years brings a deepening realisation of our own uniqueness, a perception of the truth that we have been created unparalleled, the only one of our kind. The task of these years is to guide this distinctiveness towards authenticity; to integrate with reverence and respect the various parts of the psyche, the body and its needs, the emotions and sexuality, into an integral person. From the free and loving acceptance of that personhood will spring the spiritual perspective which becomes ours at this moment of life.

Spirituality may be seen as the response of the whole person to God, as he calls, gifts and graces us. It is, therefore, a very individual thing, a relationship offered by God and responded to by each one out of his or her uniqueness. It is radical, has to do with roots, roots which are anchored deep in our own life story. It also implies a rootedness in God from whom is drawn the life which flows through our being. These two elements, human life in all its dimensions, and the divine life breathed into us, are the important strands which underlie any spirituality.

We find in our human histories a personal revelation of God as he wishes to make himself known to each one. There he shows what he wants our relationship with him to be. The events of life give to the spirituality of each person a particular distinctive quality, yet these may be influenced and coloured by the spiritual tradition of others, whether it be an Ignatius, a Catherine of Sienna or a Francis of Assisi.

Because we live and respond to God in a particular world culture, it, too, must be expected to influence this response to some degree. Christian spirituality is in dialogue with the times in which we live and cannot be isolated from or lived outside this culture. So there has been a change in emphasis throughout the centuries from a stress on community in the early church, and later on asceticism, to a spirituality focused on incarnation and creation in the present day.

It is this last which can speak very relevantly in the second half of life. Creation-centred spirituality highlights the sacredness of all life and the responsibility of mature men and women to tend and nurture it, to be its 'stewards', enhancing rather than destroying it. They are 'the mind and heart of the planet'[1] called to discover the meaning and significance of this world through their awareness and their power of reflection. Thomas Berry, and before him Teilhard de Chardin, speak of the human as 'that being in whom the universe activates, reflects upon, and celebrates itself in conscious self-awareness'.[2] Co-creators with God, humankind transforms cosmic energy into a life-giving, healing force, awakening the earth and its people to their own 'profusion of beauty and of being'.[3]

For each one, the greatest of God's gifts is, however,

his or her own individual existence which must be respected and cared for so that it can reach its future potential and ultimate fulfilment. But this can only be attained by turning out towards others and the universe in service and in love. To reverence life is to recognise it as blessing, within which there are limits, but these limits can yield a rich source of new growth. Like Augustine, we come to see our lives in totality and totally graced.

Spiritual development, like that of the psyche or of sexuality, has long been recognised as occurring in a definite pattern. A series of stages has been described variously by different theologians. St John of the Cross, who combined a profound sense of psychology with his theological approach, is one of the clearest and best known exponents of such development. Not only a great mystic himself, he was also a brilliant theologian and an eminent poet, with a gift of expression which enabled him to communicate to others much of his own experience of God. He depicted three well-defined phases, each of which is prepared for by a period of transition or crisis known as a conversion. This description is not simply a way for the mystic: all go through these stages in varying degrees of intensity.

The first conversion, that of the beginner, he described as a prelude to a time of reconciliation and of sensible consolation in our relating to God. This has been called the Purgative Way. The tendency to settle in the relative peace of this stage is shattered by the onset of the second conversion, known also as the Dark Night of the Senses, a time of dryness and a waning of the consolation which had previously meant so much. Most of the suffering of this transition consists in the inability to find God as before. Gradually a detachment from the things of sense takes place and a new knowledge of God emerges. A time of contemplation, rather than of discursive prayer, marks the Way of the Proficient, or the Illuminative Way. In its turn this, too, is disrupted by the third and most severe of the conversions, the Dark Night of the Spirit. Here a stripping of what hinders union with God takes place and is usually accompanied by aridity, desolation and near despair.

It is not difficult to see the analogy between the suffering of this period and that which occurs during the mid-life crisis when one must open up to God in a courageous act of self-surrender. Just as it is possible to become entrapped in the crisis of mid-life and never move beyond it, so many are unable to take the step of total surrender necessary to enter the Way of the Perfect, the Unitive Way, that is the final stage of union with God.

Whether we travel the *via negativa* of St John of the Cross which stresses the transcendence of God and the stripping of self, or the *via positiva* which is concerned more with his immanence in creation and our right use and respect of created things, depends much upon temperament. But whichever the way, a similar developmental pattern is evident, bringing about a transformation in the spiritual life.

St Teresa of Avila described this same journey in story form as a pilgrimage through six mansions or dwelling places of the Interior Castle to the seventh and central one. Here union with God is completed. Her description of the passage through the third mansion corresponds in many ways with that experienced during the mid-life crisis. Her fourth dwelling place, where God is met in the prayer of recollection and of quiet, marks the beginning of the individuation process of the second half of life.

In these ways two doctors of the church describe the normal passage taken in the search for a closer relationship with God. It is the complex changes occurring in the psyche during the second half of life which facilitate this movement. In becoming more integrated, more fully human, we increase the capacity for the spiritual. Though by no means identical, psychology and spirituality are closely linked, the one enabling the other. How then do the changes occurring during the middle years promote our spiritual development and lead to a deeper intimacy with God?

The emerging power of interiority in early mid-life allows us to enter our inner world in a new way, to journey within and to explore previously unknown realms. It is here that we discover a new and paradoxical truth: that it is in letting go that we come into possession. Here, too, we meet God at a depth we could not reach earlier in life, though this meeting may be shrouded in darkness. We can open ourselves to a source of love and power with faith that has matured through its time of trial, and can find in the emergent Self the mystery that it is within this that the Father makes his home.

This new capacity to ponder at depth leads one to get in touch with the whole of life in an ego-less reflection. If time is taken to reflect in prayer on life's experiences, we will hear God's word uttered in a revelation of himself that is entirely personal to each one.

Life is God's gift and it comes enfolded in the happenings of every day. To unwrap and discover that gift fully means to explore those events, to appreciate what they disclose of God's love and his hopes for us. This personal revelation of himself through the circumstances of life speaks of the particular friendship he wishes to have with each one. Just as it was in their story that the people of Israel learnt that they were to be a chosen people, so it is in each one's own story that his or her calling is revealed.

This 'scripture' of our lives, God speaking to us even as he spoke to Moses 'as a man speaks to his friend' (Exodus 33:11), brings an understanding of the theme of our spirituality. Paul, as he reflected on what had happened to him since Damascus, became aware that it was only as he gave over his own strength and power that the Lord could freely work in him, 'for it is when I am weak that I am strong' (2 Corinthians 12:10). In the same way Elizabeth of the Trinity discovered her call to praise the glory of God, and Thérèse of Lisieux to walk the way of littleness.

Just as we value the word spoken in the scripture of the bible, so we come to an appreciation of God's word discovered in the scripture of life, and learn to pray with that text too. Attentive to the message spoken through the prophet Isaiah we can be assured of its truth: 'As the rain and the snow come down from the heavens and do not return without watering the earth, making it yield and giving growth . . . so the word that goes from my mouth does not return to me empty, without . . . succeeding in what it was sent to do.' (Isaiah 55:10-11). We are empowered through our own salvation history to respond to the God who accompanies us on life's journey, sure that his word will succeed in what it was sent to do for us also.

The mid-life crisis, an occasion of special openness to God, can nevertheless be experienced as a time when all sense of relatedness is lost. The suffering may be intense as, engulfed in a cloud of darkness, we become lost in the bewildering turmoil which results. Faced with the negative side of the 'shadow' we are dismayed by what becomes evident there. Yet it is only in the acceptance of sinfulness and limitation that wholeness can finally be attained.

Maria Boulding makes clear that 'the backdrop to creation, both the old creation and the new, is chaos'.[4]

This is the case so often as we stand on the threshold of the second half of life unaware, as yet, of its richness and creativity.

For some, this time of chaos may reveal itself simply as a re-evaluation of life, a reflection on the limits of what has been achieved and an acceptance of this in truth; a recognition of dependency, in humility and trust. It may entail a re-examination of an original calling and perhaps a stronger commitment as that call is once more confirmed. Again, such evaluation may lead to listening in another direction and a consequent change in orientation. All this can take place without too much disruption in an otherwise busy and satisfying career.

However, there are others who experience a far more painful transition in the middle years and this is reflected in their spiritual life. They can be faced with a bewildering change for which they can see no apparent cause. Whereas up until now prayer has brought peace and a certain measure of consolation, suddenly God seems to withdraw leaving them in darkness and uncertainty. Images which previously spoke to them become empty and meaningless. The pain of this apparent loss can be severe and the loneliness and sense of emptiness frightening. As a married woman entering her forties confessed: 'I am almost afraid of trying to pray now as God seems to have deserted me and I feel only the agony of a terrible void in place of the closeness that used to be there.'

Acutely aware of limitations, poverty and weakness, many seem unable to find the God for whom they are longing, sometimes even without knowing it. This in itself can be part of the suffering. No longer sensing the need or desire for him, they are enveloped in a barren winter of the spirit.

There is often a strong temptation to discontinue the struggle, as the effort to go on seems too painful. The lesson of Gethsemane then becomes central. It is only by following Christ in an acceptance of desolation, in staying with the distress, that they can hope to rise with him to a new quality of spiritual life.

The re-evaluation of life's journey may confront us with our own poverty, brokenness and sinfulness, even with what appears as our rottenness. At such times it can help to recall that the God we are searching for is not a God of the rich and the powerful but one who was drawn in a special way to the *anawim*, the little ones, of Israel; one who showed a particular predilection for the poor and the outcasts, who did not shrink from embracing the leper but found his joy in searching out the lost and rejected ones of the land. A growing acceptance of fragility and poverty of heart will reveal something of what Paul discovered when he spoke of weakness as 'his special boast' since because of it 'the power of Christ' could reveal itself in him. (2 Corinthians 12:9)

The sense of loss which is at the heart of all crisis, and no less that of mid-life, can propel us into a conviction of total uselessness and emptiness. We are useless because we are no longer in control, empty because we have lost our self-determination. Like Peter, we are being asked to be willing to be 'taken where you would rather not go'. (John 21:18) This is often the moment of coming to an awareness of the ways in which we have attempted in the past to control God, to expect him to follow the paths we saw best, to grant those things we judged essential. Now it is that the Lord speaks to us in the strong but tender words once addressed to Israel:

For I knew you to be obstinate,
your neck an iron bar ...
For the sake of my name I deferred
my anger ...
And now I have put you in the fire
like silver,
I have tested you in the furnace of
distress ...
I, Yahweh, your God, teach you
what is good for you,
I lead you the way you must go.

(Isaiah 48:4, 9–11, 17)

To let go of ego-centredness, and the countless idols we have built for ourselves is the challenge he calls us to now. Only then will we be led through the darkness of loss and the desert of uncertainty, knowing that both are 'the place of God's closeness and care'.[5]

The parable of the grain of wheat (John 12:24) speaks profoundly to the mid-lifer. If full fruitfulness is to be found, then the wheat grain must fall into the earth and die to its own way of living so that it can finally yield a rich harvest. The disintegration of so much that seemed good in the first half of life must take place before we can reach out to take hold of the wealth that lies ahead. Our level of trust must be re-worked to allow for the handing over of the control of our lives, knowing that we are being led to a new vitality by one who is tender and compassionate, rich in his mercy and forgiveness. In an unpublished poem entitled 'Unless the Seed ...', a religious at mid-life gave expression to the struggle with darkness and confusion which threatened to crush the faint glow of hope that she held in her heart.

How can the seed tell
Whether the earth is grave or
womb?
Can it know from the confines
Of its narrow tomb
The springing birth of tomorrow?

But my heart knows.
It feels the stirring of life
Sown in the cold clay of my
being.
Seed of love
Begin your strife.
Reach up to greet,
Through the coiled hard earth of
my heart,
The sun's heat, love's life-bringing
breath.

He who loses his life for my
sake . . .
But this is death!
How can life break
Out of such still cold clay,
self-slime?

Yet I know in whom I have
believed.
It is time to entrust vitality to the
clay.
Unless the seed . . . there is no
other way.
Break the hard earth
With the green shoots of your
strong meekness.
He who knows all can do all
And most with our weakness.

Drop your defences, shed your
dry shell,
Seed of love in my deep heart's
being.
This shrivelled emptiness
Is prelude to a fuller being.
He who alone gives fruitfulness
He will bring you to birth, seed of
love
Struggling to express the
inexpressible
Out of this dark earth.

Who can tell if you will succeed?
Love is the answer, love's seed,
'And all shall be well'.[6]

It is in coming to an acceptance of ourselves as weak and sinful, limited and constantly failing, that we reach openness to a God who wants nothing more than the gift of ourselves as we are. It is he who will become our strength, will fill our emptiness and bring healing to our sinfulness, he who will lead us through a sense of our vulnerability to a wellspring of wisdom, empathy and compassion. The pain experienced will become a source of sensitivity to those who suffer; acknowledgement of weakness will bring tolerance of the fragility of others and a willingness to help them support the burden of their existence.

The years of mid-life are, too, a time of significant spiritual healing. Not only is there need to be healed of sinfulness but there is a growing awareness of the hurt inflicted by others in the course of life's journey. With the expansion of consciousness, emphasised by Jung, much that was thought to be buried and forgotten begins to surface. Memories return of incidents in which one has been damaged, rejected or angered.

These may not emerge first as recalled events but rather as pain re-experienced when slighted, or an insupportable rage at something which in itself seems trivial. The depth of the pain or the extent of the anger shows that the source is something beyond the present incident. To permit oneself to feel these emotions and to sit with them will often bring to mind a time of hurt or unjust treatment in the past, possibly even in childhood. This memory, like a deep-festering wound, may have lain hidden for many years. As it comes back now, it is crying out to be remembered and reconciled. It was Henri Nouwen who pointed out that 'there is no hope for the future when the past remains unconfessed, unreceived and misunderstood'.[7]

The prayer of healing can, therefore, play a vital part in the spirituality of mid-life. There is a temptation to push back the memory into the unconscious in the hope that forgetting it again will ease the pain. But this is not the case. Hidden though it is, it will continue to colour experience, to deepen vulnerability or intensify anger. Brought to a healing it can become a source of enrichment and often a cause of profound joy. This was evident in the case of a marriage brought close to disaster by the damage done to both partners in childhood. As husband and wife came to accept their past and to bring it to healing in prayer a strong bond of understanding grew up between them resulting in a serenity and a deep happiness that had not existed in their marriage before.

To bring a past event to healing in this way means that, in prayer, the pain, shame, anger or bitterness involved, is re-experienced. It is not enough simply to think about these emotions. They must be felt again, accepted and acknowledged. Then the Lord can touch the place of one's pain in the same way as he laid his hands on the woundedness and brokenness of so many men and women throughout the length and breadth of Palestine. Stay with that touch until the feeling drains away and is replaced by an acceptance and peace.

Again the hurt may be imaged, appearing for example as a great load, a sharp sword or a threatening cloud. In prayer, this can be placed in the Lord's hands and watched as he gradually transforms it. For one person the sense of rejection, which had weighed on him since childhood, was perceived as a heavy stone. As he placed this in the hands of Jesus in imagery, the stone slowly began to shrink until he saw only a piece of shining black coal. Gradually, as he watched, it was transformed into the brilliance of diamond. He realised then that, for the first time, he could truly feel for others who had suffered something similar to himself. This, for someone who was both counsellor and spiritual director, added a new quality to his being with others. Not only was his pain gone but he had acquired a precious gift to use in his ministry.

Healing of memories can take many forms and it sometimes requires several months, or even years, of such prayer before acceptance and peace is attained. The healing is not completed, however, until forgiveness of those responsible for the injury, or of oneself if necessary, is reached. Once this has taken place there is a sense of freedom, even of joy, and what was a cause of suffering becomes a source of gratitude.

At times an incident may appear to be healed, only to re-emerge later with a further revelation of the pain from a deeper level of the unconscious. This must again be brought to prayer until finally all the ramifications have been touched and healed.

Memories of happier times when others have loved, praised or rejoiced with us, or we have gone out to another in this way, can also be reflected on in prayer. The prayer of reminiscence can be strengthening and reassuring during the middle years when many are, perhaps, doubting their self-worth or loveableness. It, too, should involve a re-experiencing of the joy, the warmth or the goodness of these times. This prayer can also bring with it a deep sense of gratitude for the goodness of life. Gratitude for gifts received is a powerful means of drawing us out of ourselves, especially in times of feeling lost, helpless or depressed.

The second half of life is also a time of expanding the capacity for intimacy as a depth of self-awareness, not possible before, is reached. This empowers us to give ourselves more completely to another in love. It is reflected in the way we meet God as well as in our relations with others. No longer is the expression of love so urgent. It becomes more open, more receptive, less anxious to control. Sexual intimacy at this stage of life not only mirrors the outpouring of love in the Godhead but can open the couple to receive that divine love, together with the human, and experience something of its transforming power in their lives.

As the turmoil and confusion of crisis is left behind the growing power of intimacy leads to a transformation in our prayer. Union with God is expressed wordlessly: we can be still in his presence, wanting nothing more than to be there. This prayer of quiet, a tranquil breathing in of love, of sureness of God's closeness though it may not be felt, brings with it a new found peace. It grows out of the darkness, the giving over of self which is a necessary prelude to God's becoming truly central in our lives. Prayer now becomes more a listening, an awareness of God's action within. No longer do we seek so urgently for signs of his presence or feel so in need of re-assurance that what we are doing, or not doing, is right. Faith assures us that he is there, a loving presence taking over our lives, and teaching that it is more important to be open to his love than to give expression to our own.

This transformation is revealed also in our approach to the world and the society in which we live. There can be a gradual discovery and acquisition of 'the mind of Christ', perceiving world situations through his eyes, being compassionate to those who suffer with the compassion of his heart, and developing a more contemplative outlook on life.

The years of middle adulthood are indeed a time of paschal mystery, a passing-over from a life of involvement in outer things to one in which the wealth hidden within is discovered. This is accompanied by a dying of much which was held precious in earlier years, with the struggle and pain involved. Only in this way can new life be attained.

For many, it is an occasion of deep spiritual conversion, not in the sense of transferring religious affiliation, but in the profound and radical change which occurs in their relationship with God. It is a time when new dimensions become apparent in old truths and we are gradually released into the freedom of the sons and daughters of the Father. Just as those who lived through the passion, death and resurrection of Jesus were transformed by the experience, so too are we. The Peter of the post-resurrection Tiberias was a very different person from the ardent fisherman who plied those seas three years previously. Deepened and matured by pain and tested in the fire of ultimate failure in his betrayal, he was now prepared to accept the burden of leadership and to assume the care of the new-born church.

These years mark for most the transition from what

the Whiteheads describe as the discipleship of the young adult to the stewardship which comes with maturity.[8] To be 'steward' means to assume a responsibility for the welfare of the persons and things of this world, to become generative. Religious generativity is at the very heart of our stewardship. It is the desire to hand on to others the gift that we have received, a knowledge of truth and a faith that has become precious to us. But to be generative means also to be detached, to be sufficiently flexible to embrace new ideas, new ways of acting. Generativity speaks of that very difficult combination of caring so much that we want to give life and hope to those who follow us, while, at the same time, being detached to the extent that we can let go and allow others to find their own maturity.

We have only to look at the generativity of Jesus to learn how this can be done. In his dealings with his closest friends he moulded them gently but firmly into the leaders he wished them to be, then placed in their keeping the legacy he had for the world: 'I have given them the teaching you have given me.' (John 17:18) He shared with them his experience of God as 'Abba', a loving Father, and left them the prayer that would bring to coming generations a new understanding of their creator. The final gift of his life in love was accompanied by the invitation to each of his followers to lay down their lives for the sake of others. For we cannot be givers of life until we have consented to die to ourselves, as he did, with all the pain that is involved. The same message was reiterated again after his resurrection. 'Do you love me?' (John 21:15) he asked Peter three times and each time in response to his reply urged him to turn outward to care for others. 'Do not cling,' he told Mary Magdalene, 'but go to my people and tell them I am risen.' (John 20:17) Only after the time of their testing were they commissioned to spread the Good News.

Mid-life spirituality consists then of listening to God's invitation spoken from the darkness and near despair of crisis. It means allowing oneself to be stripped of self-determination, discovering and accepting weakness and emptiness and enduring the agonising pain of loss. Then the woman and man in the middle years will be prepared to respond to the summons to generative leadership in the church and in society, sure that the power and strength needed will be given them.

Rainer Maria Rilke expresses a little of what Paul spoke of when he referred to the Corinthians, and through them to each one, as earthenware vessels: empty only that they might be filled with the 'overwhelming power' of God. (2 Corinthians 4:7)

It is hard, the descent to God, but see
You're plying your empty vessels in distraction,
When to be child, girl, woman's suddenly
enough to give him endless satisfaction.

He is the water: you need only mould
the cup out of two hands extended yonder:
and, if you kneel as well — why then he'll squander,
and pass all your capacity to hold.[9]

♦ ♦ ♦

Chapter • 11

THE CHALLENGE OF AGEING

Coming to terms with the decline or loss of mid-life powers, readies us to move into the last season of life. This has an excitement and a beauty all its own, but one sometimes difficult to perceive at first.

With the progression from middle to late adulthood somewhere in the sixties, we are faced again with the pain of crisis. This is frequently associated with the traumas of adjusting to a new life-style following on retirement or illness. Again, the sudden realisation that death may not be too far removed can initiate a time of struggle and unrest. It is in this period of transition that order is imperceptibly re-established out of the turmoil and chaos and a further restructuring of the personality takes place.

For most, there is not a sudden onset to ageing. It is something that physical, and possibly mental, changes gradually bring to awareness. Levinson speaks of two phases of this final developmental period, Late Adulthood from about sixty to eighty-five and Late Late Adulthood which covers the completion of life's journey. A progressive stoop, an aching joint, or a lessening ability to negotiate the hills may all be indicators that age is catching up. As Robert Butler, a renowned geriatric specialist, points out: 'Old age is a period of rapid, profound and multiple changes of varying intensities ... which influence subjective experience, behaviour and adaptation.'[1] However, many of these changes may not be age-specific but rather the result of illness or of some social factor. 'How come?' said one eighty-six-year-old when told his aching knee was due to ageing. 'I have another just as old and it's as good as new.'

The coming of senescence, a gentler term than ageing, is usually the time to hand over to younger generations the many responsibilities assumed in mid-life, to quit the centre stage, and leave the throne of power to settle for the seat of wisdom. Although many ageing men and women still play an important role in business, politics and the intellectual world, bringing to it the fruit of their experience, for most there is a call to reduce the heavy burden of involvement. Late Adulthood remains a time of fulfilment but in a different relationship to society and to oneself. It is not always easy to face this change.

Deprived of an active role in a school or hospital community, many older religious women and men have sought out the needy in other areas. One discovered the plight of children at risk in violent home situations and devoted her time and considerable energy in travelling to comfort a two-year-old in a city hospital. He was suffering from the effects of violence from a mother over-stressed by the problems in her own life. After years of patient backing from his 'grandmother', this now teenage boy still turns to her for the encouragement he needs.

To age graciously is perhaps one of the most difficult of life's tasks for those who live in a western society. In many oriental cultures, the respect given to the mature aged, especially in the past, confirmed their value to the population as a whole. It made growing old not only acceptable but also an event to be looked forward to with pride. The insights and experience of the aged were a source of wisdom and inspiration for every generation. Elders were surrounded with deference and esteem, and ministered to with honour and affection. To the western world, however, to be old is, for the most part, to be regarded as useless, unattractive and unwanted. It is little wonder, then, that age is often denied and attempts are made with paints and powders, and even cosmetic surgery, to camouflage the wear and tear of passing years.

For women especially, age brings depreciation in the eyes of many, a fact exploited by the numerous producers of beauty products and 'age-controlling' creams. Whereas the lined and wrinkled face speaks of character and nobility in the man, the white hair of dignity and distinction, in the woman they are thought of as undesirable accretions of the years. Women grow old, men become distinguished, but even they must face a loss of consequence in their later years. Is growing old, then, nothing more than a negation of all we have striven for in life?

The challenge of ageing well is a call to understand that, whereas youth may be a gift of nature, age is indeed a work of art. It cannot be achieved without the necessary stripping and sculpting which will finally reveal the essential beauty lying within each one. Rarely do we pause to appreciate what is offered to those who, in God's Providence, are destined to live out the full span of life. No matter how endowed or virtuous the young are, there is something beyond their reach which can only be grasped by those gifted with the fullness of years. They alone can hope to reach that integrity, that full comprehension of the meaning of life, which remains concealed from those who have not yet acquired the wisdom of the aged. In this continued growth to wholeness lies the grace of ageing.

In a recent interview given to the *New York Times* in her eighty-sixth year, Joan Erikson conceded: 'Lots of old people don't get wise, but you don't get wise unless you age.' Their own ageing has brought to the Eriksons a further development of the understanding drawn previously from observing those who had reached integrity. Exploring the meaning of this last stage of life, Erik Erikson had found originally that these are the years during which the maturing strengths of hope, will, purpose, competence, fidelity, love and care, acquired through the course of life's journey, are forged into a comprehensive sense of wisdom.

Now, as he and his wife sat in their favourite nook in a bay window of their Cambridge home, they expanded on this theme to a young reporter, discussing the effect of the successful re-integration of each earlier phase on the ultimate development of wisdom in old age. Their own experience, and that of many whom they had followed over the years, has convinced them of the importance of 'the vital involvements necessary at each stage, from the first to the last'[2] and the re-integration of these if we are to reach full maturity and integrity in the concluding phase of the life cycle.

The coming to birth of wisdom in one's later years is then the culmination of a life-time struggle. Human interdependence, the need we each have for others, which is so necessary at this stage of life, is the fruit of a successful re-integration of the trust which first emerged from a supportive environment in the infant's earliest years. Here was laid the foundation of a hopefulness in the goodness of the universe which will flower later into a mature 'faith in being',[3] and a conviction of the concerned presence of God.

As the body begins to fail or diminish the older person must strive to maintain, as far as possible, the independence first acquired in early childhood as the strength of will grew through the acquisition of control over body functions. The right balance between healthy compliance and a sense of self-determination will result in an ability to maintain autonomy and at the same time a willingness to accept with peace a deteriorating body. When no longer able to see well enough to sew her grandchildren's clothes, one woman presented her treasured sewing machine to her daughter in a gesture revealing both autonomy and an acceptance of her diminishment.

The playfulness and creativity first developed in the preschool child is an important element in a satisfying ageing. It is the source of humour and adventurousness and leads to a re-balancing of initiative and guilt to 'temper self-interest and expansiveness with co-operation and concern for others'.[4] From this springs a certain resilience as well as an understanding and empathy with others. 'The more you know yourself, the more patience you have for what you see in others,' according to the way Joan Erikson experiences it. 'You don't have to accept what people do, but understand what leads them to it. The stance this leads to is to forgive even though you still oppose.'[5] The limitations to mobility and to sensory acuity which often accompany ageing must be countered by an initiative which renews the sense of purpose in life. To maintain the strength of purposefulness, first instilled at play, is an integral part of successful maturing.

The competence or skill developed in the child, as he or she attempts to become an effective and industrious member of society and to outweigh a feeling of inferiority, fosters a sense of humility in later life. The elder comes to accept limitations while at the same time discovering new and age-appropriate ways of learning, or sharing the knowledge and wisdom accumulated over a life time.

Identity must also be re-appraised as the old 'struggle to reconcile a sense of who they have been during their long lives with a newer, everchanging sense of who they may yet come to be in old age'.[6] Commitment to relationships with others and to the many activities which have given rise to an awareness of personal identity in earlier life is so often lost or changed during the latter period of the life cycle. It is only by integrating present involvement in society with earlier hopes, beliefs and commitments that a life-long sense of identity will come into being.

The need for intimacy in late adulthood is just as real as it was in the twenties, although the quality of closeness may have changed. 'You put such stress on passion when you're young. You learn about the value of tenderness when you grow old,' confided one woman. 'You also learn in later life not to hold: to give without hanging on; to love freely in the sense of wanting nothing in return.' Reminiscing about past intimacies can help the older person to re-integrate qualities of affection, tenderness and sexuality. Intimacy must still be balanced with the experience of aloneness which can be particularly painful if this isolation is caused by the death of a cherished partner or of a longtime friend. Closeness expressed spontaneously by touch, a kiss from a son or daughter, a hug from a friend, can help keep alive the capacity for love in the ageing person.

Generativity, which is so closely linked with wisdom, most frequently reveals itself in later life through two aspects — 'caritas', which Erikson takes in the broad sense of true caring for others, and 'agape', an empathic and concerned love. New ways of maintaining the generative responsibility for future generations developed in the middle years must be found if the older person is to resist the pull to self-absorption. This becomes more pressing as so many avenues of expressing this concern are closed off by failing health or isolation. The ageing adult is challenged to accept care from others in a way that is in itself caring, and to integrate concern for the outside world and attention to the inner world, without becoming egotistic or self-centred.

It is only the person who has emerged caring and concerned from the crisis of generativity at mid-life, and anxious in some way to enhance the lives of others, who will achieve the strength of wisdom.

As one struggles in the later years to bring into balance 'the life-long sense of trustworthy wholeness and the opposing sense of bleak fragmentation',[7] much will depend on the situation in which each is placed. Even in this final stage the environment plays a critical role in who we eventually become. Surrounded by acceptance and love, the struggle to prevent despair overwhelming the sense of integrity is not so difficult. Rejected or unwanted by society, it is hard to hold on to a faith and trust in others, a sense of identity as a worthwhile contributor, or the ability to love and be involved with others. Who has not seen the elderly person living alone or perhaps confined, for some good reason, to an institution in which no one has time or care for him or her? The fight to maintain dignity and a sense of worth may well give way to isolation, self-occupation and despair.

As the end of life's journey draws near each one is confronted with the basic questions: Who am I? Have I become the person I was created to be? Am I now my unique, authentic self? The story is told of the rabbi, Susya, who became restless and disturbed as death approached. Those standing around his bed enquired if he was worried that the Lord might enquire why he had not become another Moses. 'No,' he replied, 'my worry is that he will find that I have not yet become completely Susya.' His anxiety was that he may not have reached that unique integrity of personality which he alone could attain.

The successful movement towards integrity requires coming to terms with choices made and accepting them now as an inevitable part of life. These have all been responsible for making us the persons we have become. Perhaps with other options there would have been a difference but now our paths have been determined. The time has come to 'accept one's own and only life cycle and the people who have become significant to it as something that had to be and that, by necessity, permitted of no substitutions'.[8] We may, with Robert Frost, sigh for 'The Road Not Taken' but we know that our destiny now lies on the one 'having perhaps the better claim'.

Two roads diverged in a wood,
and I —
I took the one less travelled by,
And that has made all the
difference.[9]

There may still be areas in our lives in need of healing, of forgiveness, of re-working in some way and all this must be attended to. When it is completed a sense of the 'givenness' of it all can be reached, an ability to accept what has been without being overwhelmed by a sense of failure, of regret or disgust. This movement to acceptance of life as it has been leads to integrity which is the fruit of full human maturity. Inspired by ripened wisdom, new joy and gladness that we are as we are will liberate us more and more from regrets and condemnations. Those who have harmed us or altered the pattern of our lives can be forgiven. Parents are no longer the scapegoats, the reason for our failure. A mature love and respect for those who formed us blossoms as we learn to take responsibility for ourselves; learn, too, to appreciate even the hardships which have brought a certain richness into life.

It is through this self-acceptance and the acceptance of the past that we arrive at a broader conceptualisation of the meaning of life itself and of our own life in particular. Personal failures are matched with personal success, self-reproach gives way to a sense of self-esteem, and death can then be approached with calm serenity.

Jung, in speaking of this time of life's afternoon writes: 'Ageing people should know that their lives are not mounting [as the sun] and unfolding, but that an inexorable inner process forces the contraction of life. For a young person it is almost a sin — and certainly a danger — to be too much occupied with himself; but for the ageing person it is a duty and a necessity to give serious attention to himself. After having lavished its light on the world, the sun withdraws its rays in order to illumine the self.'[10]

This intensification of the movement from outer to inner world interests, leads to a meeting with a further archetype, that of the old man or woman within.

Archetypes, as was seen earlier, are those abiding patterns in the psyche which, once embraced, energise the journey to individuation. They are encountered most clearly in dreams or projections and met in art, literature or myths which deeply move or maybe even terrify us. When dealing with the integration of the anima and animus, one of the tasks of mid-life individuation, we recognised that it is often the negative or dark side of the archetype which first becomes evident. This less desirable aspect must be acknowledged and accepted if we are to discover its richer, brighter side. This is why we are so often struck initially by the ugliness of ageing, the loss of power, of appearance and of all that seems loveable in us.

Little wonder then that the temptation is there to reject this emerging image from the psyche. But if ageing is denied and not admitted into consciousness, there will be a strong reaction in the face of evidence of age in those around us. This is an obvious projection. One woman spoke of feeling profoundly disturbed each time she walked into the diningroom of a retirement village. As she saw there the old and furrowed faces of those who sat and waited to be served, something inside her seemed to cry out in resistance. She realised then that she was denying her own ageing, that unless she could accept this fact it would continue to haunt her. Only by admitting its reality into consciousness could she regain her peace of mind. Once acknowledged and accepted, her age became a welcomed part of life. By denying the ageing woman or man in us, we allow ourselves to be possessed by the negative aspect of the archetype, becoming bitter, querulous, complaining or censorius. But when the reality of advancing years is invited into consciousness, its distinctive beauty is discovered. The ugliness of ageing, the negative side of the archetype, gives way to reveal the wise old man or old woman in our lives, the person we are striving to become. A transformation is then experienced, a rebirth of the personality.

This was clearly perceived by Rhonda in a dream: 'I saw an older woman dressed in long, flowing robes, surrounded by a group similarly dressed and talking quietly together. Suddenly the older woman seemed in some way to diminish. I could not see exactly what was happening as the others gathered close around her as if to hide what was taking place. Then a voice said clearly: "This is becoming difficult for the sisters, but they are trying to be loving." With that a stream of water poured from the woman's hands and body as if she was dissolving and she was carried out of sight. Then the other women knelt and with great reverence kissed the saturated ground where she had stood. I felt deeply moved and somehow full of awe. The scene shifted and the woman reappeared, dancing, transformed and younger in appearance. Love and joy radiated from her. I found myself exclaiming: "This is truly life."'

The dreamer interpreted her dream as speaking of the need to love and revere her failing body. She must accept the many losses age was bringing if she were to gain the freedom, joy and hope that could well be hers. The sense of awe felt in the dream spoke to her of a deep spiritual surrender, a letting go.

All must face the fact of ageing but there will be a fundamental difference between the one who resists this destiny holding firmly to the past, and the one who welcomes it as an inevitable passage to a fuller life.

Jung wrote very little about these last years of life, perhaps because for him they were no more than a continuation of the process of individuation already begun. The archetype of the old man or woman is but one of 'the many aspects of unreconciled multiplicity in us'.[11] the light and the dark, the yin and the yang. We will continue until life's end to discover from the unconscious new aspects of ourselves as we draw nearer to full self-possession and the wisdom which is the fruit of years.

One of the gravest fears about the losses of these later years is that they will include a serious decline in intellectual ability and a deprivation of mental powers. But this is rarely the case. It is not the normal concomitant of ageing. Research assures us that the average intelligence quotient of the aged is even higher than that among the young or middle-aged. It would appear to be a matter of the survival of the fittest. In research carried out at the University of Queensland between 1960 and 1980, it soon became apparent 'that the geriatric disablement and mental deterioration of a certain proportion of the elderly had been generalised to the whole gerontological scene, because too little research had been focused upon normal ageing processes'.[12] The finding showed that the decrement was not a matter of serious concern before the age of eighty when it amounted to an average annual loss of 2 per cent, and by ninety of 2.72 per cent. Some subjects showed no loss at all after fifteen years, while the ratings of a few revealed a slight improvement.

One factor which accelerates deterioration is the lack of stimulation and the disuse of intellectual powers. For this reason it is important to stimulate the mind and to keep mentally alive. 'I set before you life or death. Choose life, then,' (Deuteronomy 30:19) was the invitation issued to the people of Israel as they prepared to enter the promised land, and the same challenge comes to those who are leaving youth behind. They can choose to remain intellectually alert, to sustain mental agility, or can be satisfied with opting for death and sinking into mental stagnation. To maintain an interest in current affairs with a healthy curiosity in what goes on in the world is to remain vital and alert in mind. Television, reading, courses in adult education and a countless variety of games can act as stimulants to mental processes. 'I have made a resolution to keep my community informed of what is happening in the world,' declared one seventy-eight-year-old religious. 'In this way we won't get out of touch.' She followed every news commentary and read widely until she became one of the best informed people I have ever met. Another took out a subscription to a scientific journal at ninety to keep in touch with current theories.

Dr Elsie Harwood has provided ample evidence that older people can benefit greatly from opportunities for learning and for acquiring further skills. 'The objective should be a level of mobility, communication, social interaction, emotional arousal, creativity, vocal exercise and, above all, mental exercises to facilitate recall, comprehension, speech and thinking generally,' she told a group of gerontologists. Not only are handcrafts, painting, gardening, games and exercises of importance, but the study of languages, of literature and history or of a musical instrument can all give a sense of achievement and help to maintain the elder's place in society. The challenge of competing with younger students at the university in no way deterred the eighty- and ninety-year-olds studying German in Dr Harwood's research programme. They found it stimulating and enjoyable as it kept them in touch with new ideas and interests. One eighty-nine-year-old had to confess to failing to do his homework for two weeks as he had been tinkering with the engine of the 1927 vintage car in which he drove himself to the university to sit for his exam. Others of a similar age group mastered the art of playing the recorder, competing favourably with their younger companions.

Not only do such activities encourage self-confidence and wider concerns. They can play a substantial role in stimulating memory and other mental faculties, while at the same time broadening the social context of life and fostering new friendships.

The right hemisphere of the brain, which is involved with perceptual and visuo-motor activities in right-handed individuals, is usually the most neglected in the aged; while verbal activity, centred in the left hemisphere, continues unabated in the majority.[13] Without overlooking the verbal capacity of the elderly, the functions of the right hemisphere can be stimulated by activities such as carpentry, model-making, tapestry, art, using patterns in knitting or crochet, music, square-dancing and similar pursuits.

To remain vitally alive and enthusiastic towards the evening of life requires that we find some appropriate way in which we can contribute to society at large. This quest becomes an important part of ageing.

As we pass through the sixties and on to the seventies much that previously gave meaning to life is lost. We are no longer in the professions or roles which enabled us to be of obvious service to others and the world. There can be a temptation to settle into a life of self-indulgence, or to abandon the struggle altogether because there seems to be no purpose left in living. Lacking adequate stimulation or motivation, many lose their self-confidence, self-esteem and dignity. The number of suicide attempts among the aged in some countries far outweighs those of any earlier age group and, as Alfons Deeken[14] points out, most of these prove successful. The realisation that there is no longer any need for what we can contribute to our previous field of work or to society in general can be a frightening one. It may well lead to deep depression and a serious loss of self-respect.

The need to be needed or to have some purpose in life is fundamental to the human person. It becomes an important task of later life to discover areas where our services are required or in which we can contribute in some small way.

Mandatory retirement no longer spells a necessary end to active involvement or a time of inertia and of boredom. The ageing can remain productive contributors to the social order and frequently the political arena. 'Grey Power' is becoming a force to be reckoned with in many parliamentary forums. It carries the weight of long experience and broad exposure combined with a high degree of training and expertise. The 'Gray Panthers' in the United States have made working for peace in the world one of their top priorities, conscious as they are of the destructiveness of war. Their efforts are focused also on political and educational activities to promote the welfare of the aged.

Society is enriched not only by the influence of its elders but by their active participation in a variety of areas. There are countless charitable organisations which depend on the assistance of older volunteers. Voluntary help is welcomed, too, in many community enterprises; art centres and museums readily make use of guides knowledgeable in these fields. An adventurous professional woman spent much of her retirement in archaeological digs in various parts of the country, not only contributing to the discovery of many important artefacts but at the same time broadening her knowledge of the history of her land. Another found new life in teaching handcraft to a group of prisoners. Several major cities have volunteer employment centres and offer endless opportunities to contribute skills already possessed or to acquire new ones for helping others.

In a less formal way, some elders offer their services in hospital or home visits, bringing companionship to the lonely or help to a deserted wife. One active retiree 'kept an eye on' the lawns of pensioners round about. He spent much of his week tending other people's gardens, mowing lawns and 'running up the road' to do odds and ends of shopping for those no longer as active as he. Another ageing woman learnt the intricacies of grafting because she had loved roses all her life. When her arthritic hands could no longer cut the stems, she passed on her skill to a young gardener and they worked together for long hours trading secrets.

Grandparenting is another influential role in later life. Those without children may 'adopt' grandchildren, perhaps from a nearby family in need. There seems to be a special affinity between the very young and the old. Is it because both are more simply and naturally themselves or because both can play in ways unaffected by competition or the fear of losing? Who could doubt their contribution to the younger generation after this description supplied by one small third grader: 'Grandmas are the only grownups who have got time — so everyone should have a Grandmother especially if you don't have television', or again: 'A Grandfather is a man Grandmother. He goes for walks with the boys and they talk about fishing and things like that'.[15] This relationship with the young can be one of the most rewarding and rejuvenating involvements for the ageing. For the young, it can exert a lasting influence on their lives. There is a rapport between them that has no need of words.

Both share a wonder and a wisdom which is somehow lost in the intervening years.

Many emotional wounds are healed in the children of broken families by the care and understanding that can ease the pain of separation. The grandparents may provide the one stable and reliable element in a life otherwise torn asunder by conflict and misunderstanding. It has been found that children of divorced parents adjust most rapidly with the support of the older generation. Children at risk in some families which lack this support can sometimes find the help they need in a relationship with an 'adopted' grandparent. Hospitals and children's homes often welcome an offer of such an association for the young people in their care.

There are countless ways in which the older members of society can still remain contributors. A ministry of prayer empowers us to reach out, not only to those close at hand, but to open up to world involvement. It is for each to seek out what is most meaningful and possible, even if it is as little as a single act of service every day. The time may come when all that is left to give is a smile of welcome and the serenity of one who radiates peace and joy in a world all too full of strife. When frailty takes over, the best gift we have to offer may be a gracious acceptance of the help of others.

Those who question the value of such an apparently insignificant contribution may well take heart from a simple story.

The land was parched in the lower end of the valley for this year the usual rains had failed. Waters from a distant storm high up in the mountain ranges were caught in the reservoir below, but the plains still waited, hushed to silence in their yearning for the rains to come. Two birds sat on the branch of a great oak overhanging the waters of the reservoir. 'The fields I flew past this morning,' said the swallow, 'are brown with withered grass, the crops are parched and dying. If only I could carry one drop of water to them in my beak.' 'What good is a drop of water?' said the wren. 'There is absolutely no value in a single drop of water.' With that, the last droplet from the storm rolled down a leaf surface and, with a 'plop', joined the myriad of others gathered in the reservoir below. Immediately a distant roar was heard as the sluice gates opened and a cataract of water poured into the dried river-bed below. The stream rushed on to quench the thirst of the waiting fields beyond, and bring new life to the drooping stems of corn, fresh colour to the faded flowers. 'It is indeed strange,' murmured the swallow, 'that there is absolutely no value in a single drop of water.'

A further endeavour which faces the mature adult is to remain both emotionally and intellectually flexible and willing to be exposed to change. As joints stiffen so, too, can attitudes. It is easy as one passes through the later years to become rigid, unwilling to give up 'the way it has always been'. To remain open-minded, appreciative of others' wisdom, leads to fresh creativity and a willingness to experiment with new patterns and techniques, or to be concerned with issues which previously had been all but disregarded. For the first time in life some older people find themselves engaged in campaigning for the rights of the oppressed or speaking out in defence of causes only recently espoused. The environmental movements have found inspiration and support from many who now have time to be caught up in the wonder and beauty of this planet and the fear of its possible destruction. The more mature are ready to risk offering their gifts, confident of their worth, and to develop those which may still lie dormant.

Greater tolerance of the views of others reinforces the ability to see and enter into both sides of a question or dilemma. In this way the older generation can frequently become a focal point of reconciliation, especially in the cases where their own children are concerned. Their insight and powers of discernment born from exposure to the vicissitudes of life throw fresh light on many situations.

These latter years are not, then, a time to withdraw from vital involvement in the world. The elderly have much to offer in every sphere of life, in both human and natural ecologies. This does not deny the need there is for solitude and the necessary time for reflection to gather together the threads and themes of life. It is in the consistent journey inward that we come to a possession of the authentic self and from that source draw the wisdom which is the most precious gift the elder has to offer to society. 'True human wisdom requires that a person make the long journey into the wilderness of life's joys, sufferings, possibilities, and uncanny unities amid diversity.'[16] It is not a matter of knowledge or intelligence but rather of a maturing through life's adventures and exigencies that brings to birth this wisdom of the heart.

♦ ♦ ♦

Chapter • 12

CARE OF THE AGEING BODY

As we grow to wisdom our bodies tend to become more sluggish in their functioning and less resistant to disease. It is an undisputed fact that advances in medical science have been such that most women can expect to celebrate their seventy-ninth birthday, and men their seventy-second. This, unfortunately, does not occur without an accompanying decline in youthfulness in body organs and energy reserves. Skin and body tissues take longer to heal, reactions are delayed, and hair and nails grow more slowly.

Though age of itself does not constitute an ailment, the elderly may more readily be affected by infections which would perhaps have passed unnoticed in earlier years. The body's defence or immune system begins to decline from as early as the thirties or forties and continues to do so with the advancing years. Symptoms of disease are frequently less marked in the elderly. It is not uncommon for a heart attack, a stroke or pneumonia to show no symptoms other than slight confusion. This is no indication that the disease is in any way less serious or less in need of treatment, though it does mean that it may be more readily missed or put down simply to 'old age'.

Exercise

Care of the body, an important concern at any age, becomes more so as the years pass by. Keeping oneself healthy and actively involved can be the secret of enjoying a prolonged life span. To sit in a chair, or on a park bench, all day because there is nothing left to do after retirement invites boredom and a rapid loss of vigour. Lack of exercise, and the subsequent disuse of many muscles or joints, can cause much loss of mobility and function which could otherwise be easily countered by occupations such as gardening, walking or swimming. Many eighty-year-olds are to be found happily mowing the lawn, or braving the surf, though this may not prove suitable exercise for all. Simple and appropriate exercises are readily available from community health centres for the elderly, and not so elderly, and even for those confined to wheelchairs or their beds. These can be performed to music to give added interest and freedom. Where a number of elderly people are in residence together, sessions of such exercises can provide a social context where all can enjoy their own and each other's efforts. One of the most popular social events in one nursing home was when all came together to exercise to music and many to dance. As in the case of any piece of good machinery, movement is necessary to prevent joints seizing up or muscles losing power.

Poor breathing habits is another area of concern amongst the aged. Not only is this a source of many respiratory ailments but the whole body including the brain suffers from a lowered intake of oxygen. A few good deep breaths taken regularly can expand the lungs, increasing circulation and the oxygen content of the blood. Swimming or cycling for those who can still manage it can provide an excellent means of doing this without placing stress on load-bearing joints.

Of the many forms of exercise available in this modern age, walking is perhaps the one still unsurpassed. It provides gentle movement for joints and muscles, opportunity to breathe deeply and well, and an intimacy through sight, touch and smell with the world of nature or of modern technology. Not only does it renew us physically, but walking can be a source of constant enjoyment and interest as we feel the warmth of sunshine or the bite of wind, attentive to the sound of birdcalls or the rush of traffic. The sights around us can be a source of endless wonder and can be stored in memory against the time when our feet will no longer carry us where we would like to go.

Appearance and stature

The physical changes associated with ageing are for the most part looked on with distaste. When beauty is equated with the youthful face and body, it can be difficult to recognise the altered loveliness of a face moulded by the years. 'Some people grow strikingly more beautiful in old age. Life has made them so and their faces tell a story.'[1] The serenity of those who have struggled through the trials of life and come to a source of wisdom shines out through their eyes and is reflected in their smile. The furrows and wrinkles can be seen as little more than evidence of their successful passage through the years.

Older is said to be shorter, and this is but one

indication of the change taking place in the body structure. With age muscles begin to lose their tone and skeletal modifications occur from loss of calcium from the bones, especially in women. The rounded shoulders, and perhaps humped back, are indicative of this but to a certain extent can be forestalled by exercise, a habit of erect posture and an adequate supply of calcium in the diet. Many more older women are coming to realise the need to keep fit and prevent flabbiness of muscles. These are continuing to frequent the local tennis court or swimming pool well into their sixties or seventies.

Women, too, are more inclined than men to put on weight during the second half of life, mainly as a result of a slowing-down in their metabolism. This means that calorie requirements lessen and the diet needs adjusting. Mid-life is a constant struggle with the bulge, occurring particularly around the waist and lower abdomen. Ageing often brings with it a 'drop' in weight, but not in the sense desired. Older people tend to lose fat from the upper part of the body only to redeposit it, if they are women, in the lower abdominal region, hips and thighs; and in the case of men in the upper abdomen, the 'pot' belly. 'What used to be up here,' sighed one great-grandmother, 'has now moved down there.'

Skin and hair

Not only does the skin repair itself more slowly but, in the second half of life, it begins to lose its elasticity, sagging and wrinkling as it ages. The 'bags' under the eyes which, to our horror, perhaps made their first appearance at mid-life, become more and more pronounced in later life. The skin tends to become dry and often scaly, cracking easily. It is not uncommon for a rash to appear as the result of infection invading the cracked surface. Proper care of the skin includes ensuring that it is kept soft through the use of a cream or other moisturiser where necessary. Those areas which are likely to become moist from perspiration, especially under the breasts and in the groin area, should be dried carefully and kept dry with a dusting powder. Any itching or irritation must be treated early to prevent infection becoming chronic.

Some people are awakened to the fact that they are ageing by the appearance of brown areas of pigment on their hands or other areas exposed to the sun. These are caused by alterations in the melanin in the surface of the skin due to the action of the ultraviolet light. Apart from the cosmetic effect and the teasing which sometimes accompanies their appearance, there is no need for concern about them or the brighter and more obvious liver spots. It is only if these thicken into scaly lesions, sun keratoses, that they need to be removed. Much as we love to bask in the sun, it can cause serious damage to the skin surface; to tan can form a protection against ultraviolet rays; to burn can result in keratosis, the forerunner of cancer.

Alterations in the rate of growth, the quality and colour of hair also begin during mid-life. Not only does hair begin to lose its pigment and turn grey but it also tends to thin and to become coarser in texture. In spite of what is sometimes said, this is not made worse by frequent shampooing, nor improved by constant brushing. Men are more affected than are women by thinning of the hair on the scalp, but it is also a concern for some older women and no real cure seems yet to have been found.

The growth of hair in other parts of the body, under the arms, on the legs and in the pubic area, diminishes in quantity, while facial hair may increase in women during the climacteric as a result of the growing imbalance between the oestrogen and androgen in the bloodstream. Genetic factors may also play a part in this quite normal change. Dark and coarse hair growth on the chin and upper lip is not uncommon and has nothing to do with the cosmetics or face creams which may have been used. One forty-five-year-old gave up using a particular brand of cream which she blamed for producing the first black hair on her chin. Later she resorted to electrolysis when bleaching no longer proved sufficient.

As the hair also loses its elasticity, changes occur in its capacity to curl or wave. A stronger setting lotion is usually required and the wave does not hold as long.

Sensory changes

Contrary to what is fairly generally believed, *sight* is not lost or harmed by reading in poor light, though this may cause a certain degree of stress with resulting symptoms. Older people need brighter light than those younger, because pupils decrease in size with age, allowing less light to fall on the retina. Driving at night, therefore, can be more hazardous.

The lens of the eye also undergoes a hardening process which makes accommodation more difficult: we lose some of our 'zoom' power. This starts quite early in life and becomes troublesome often for the first time during mid-life when we find our arms are not long enough to hold the book where we can read it. Glasses are needed for focusing on near objects while our distant vision may remain unchanged.

With age, there can also be increasing difficulty in distinguishing different colours. Many are not aware of this and wonder at the strange colour combinations in some older people's dress. Blues and greens become particularly difficult to differentiate. When colour is used to indicate a change in height, a step or slope, it should be bright and contrast strongly with surrounding colours.

The more serious problems in vision which can lead to blindness in the elderly are cataract, glaucoma and senile macular degeneration. All of these can be treated if they are detected soon enough. Cataract, a clouding over of the lens with a gradual loss of its transparency, is often picked up first by a blurring of vision, seeing more clearly in dimmer light, and by being readily dazzled by bright light. Cataract can be treated surgically and it is now thought better to do this before full vision is lost.

Glaucoma is characterised by increased pressure within the eye which leads to visual impairment and may finally result in blindness. Since there are few symptoms in the early stages of this disease, regular checking of the pressure within the eye-ball should be carried out if there is any loss in vision. Headaches or seeing halos around light bulbs are often indicative of glaucoma. As the pressure increases, pain is experienced in the eye and visual impairment accelerates. The earlier glaucoma is discovered and treated the less likelihood there is of permanent damage to the optic nerve.

Senile macular degeneration is the leading cause of curtailment of vision in the elderly. This diminishing and final loss of central vision is caused by either pigmentary or vascular changes in the macular area of the retina where central vision is registered. The sooner this can be detected the more hope there is of preventing further degeneration. Peripheral vision is not lost in the case of macular degeneration so that the person can still see to the sides but not directly in front of the eye.

Some older people experience the opposite: a loss of lateral vision with clearer sight being restricted to the central visual field. Retinal degeneration can also be the cause of visual loss for many diabetics.

Much is being done to assist those in the community with failing eyesight and advantage should be taken of the services offered by various societies and foundations for the blind.

There is a gradual reduction of *hearing* in the majority of the elderly. Auditory acuity is said to reach its maximum by the age of ten and from the thirties onwards there is usually some deterioration in hearing ability. Normally the higher tones are the first to be affected, so that it becomes difficult to hear the ringing of the telephone or a high-pitched alarm. Higher notes are better registered when the level of sound is low. Unfortunately most people feel that volume rather than pitch is essential, and tend to shout at older people with hearing problems. This only leads to added difficulty.

The person with diminished hearing can best follow a remark which is clearly articulated and spoken slowly in a normal or low tone of voice. As one ages, responses tend to become slower. A repeated question before one has time to work out a response only hinders the ability to reply.

Hearing aids are improving constantly and should be readily available to anyone with a hearing defect.

Both the senses of *taste* and *smell* tend to decline in later years and to require greater stimulation to register clearly. For this reason the older person may tend to eat too highly spiced dishes which can be difficult to digest. Sugar and salt consumption may tend to increase. As the sense of smell deteriorates, older people should ensure that food is not tainted, or that the gas is turned off. It is important to be aware, too, that body odours which can be offensive to others may be overlooked, so particular care with hygiene should be taken and clothing be kept clean, especially in the case of any urinary leakage or slight incontinence.

Just as *touch* is becoming recognised as particularly important to the young, so we must acknowledge its significance to the elderly. We all need to be touched or held by those who love us and this can be especially marked in an older person who has perhaps lost most close relationships. To put a hand on the shoulder or arm of an elderly person communicates a sense of affection and of his or her self-worth which is so often being doubted. Similarly a gentle touch or pat from an older person shows the warmth of their affection.

Changes in the ageing skin surface also leaves it less sensitive. Older people do not feel pain through touch as readily as before, so they should take care to see that they do not injure or burn themselves unwittingly, or that a skin lesion which they do not feel as painful receives adequate care and treatment.

Teeth and dentures

Unfortunately for many teeth seem to wear out before the rest of the human frame, consequently old age finds them with very few of their own left. Without teeth a person cannot eat properly, speak clearly or even kiss with warmth.

Where dentures are necessary it is essential that they fit well to ensure comfort and proper nourishment. They may need to be renewed, or at least readjusted, as the gums shrink with age. So often elderly people's dentures remain in the drawer or float in a glass because they can no longer be worn with comfort. One old person literally starved herself because she felt 'death was too close now to waste money on myself. The children need all I can leave them'. Her difficulty was not the cost of food but rather the fact that she could no longer chew it, and did not want to spend money on new dentures. Once persuaded that it was all right to do so, her whole life changed and she continued to live for several more years, 'getting her money's worth'.

Lesions to the gums frequently result from ill-fitting dentures and can cause great discomfort. Regular visits to the dentist are necessary as the jaw shape can also alter in the latter years.

Feet

Another part of the body which requires particular attention in the second half of life are the feet. This is especially important for those suffering from diabetes, arthritis or vascular disease. Circulatory disorders can give rise to lack of adequate blood supply, especially in the toes, thus resulting in tissue destruction and possibly gangrene. Any areas of discolouration on the feet should always be reported to the doctor.

Many falls and fractured bones are caused by poorly fitting or down-at-the-heel footwear. Soft slippers may be comfortable to use around the house but they do not give the support needed to arches of the feet or to the ankles. Well-fitting, and if need be, made-to-measurement shoes can revolutionise a person's existence. As someone said: 'If you can change a person's feet, you can change their lives.'

Regular visits to the podiatrist who will trim nails or remove callouses or corns will ensure continued mobility and comfort. There are many podiatrists who are willing to make home-calls for those who are house-bound or have difficulty in getting to the city.

Feet should be bathed daily and carefully wiped especially between the toes. Fungal infections, such as athlete's foot, readily develop in the moister areas of the feet particularly if there is a crack in the skin surface. This can give rise to uncomfortable itching and raw and painful areas as the soggy white skin is rubbed off. These infections should be treated early as the more chronic they become, the more difficult they are to cure.

Swelling of the feet or ankles may be indicative of heart or kidney disease and should be investigated professionally as soon as possible.

Bones

The brittleness of the bones in the elderly from loss of calcium, combined with poor vision, lead to frequent fractures through falls. The hip or head of the femur is one of the most common bones to suffer in this way. A frequent cause of such accidents is climbing on chairs to reach windows or cupboards rather than using graded steps. Chairs so easily slip or overbalance. The aged persons' slower reactions do not allow them to catch hold of something in time to steady themselves as a younger person might. Many women also find themselves unexpectedly hampered by a tight skirt when stepping down from a height. A simple rule: never use a chair to reach heights but have a set of steps handy.

Other common causes of accidents are tripping over electrical cords, heaters or other objects which have been left about. An older person should take care that the room is well lit and does not contain low pieces of furniture which may not be seen if peripheral vision is failing, rugs or mats which could easily slip or trip a person, extensions or rubbish containers in places where they may cause a fall. Carpet on stairs should always be firmly fixed and not so worn that a heel could catch in a tear. A simple handrail in the bathroom or shower recess and a non-slip mat will all help to avoid broken bones which take longer to knit in the older patient.

Withdrawal of calcium from the spine may give rise to the collapse of some of the vertebrae with resultant pressure on a nerve, as well as loss of height and the typical 'widow's hump'.

The digestive system

Adequate nourishment is essential for good health at every age and the failure to obtain this by some senior citizens usually has less to do with their digestive processes than with other factors. Bad eating habits are easy to fall into when one lives alone. Difficulty with chewing or loss of taste or smell all tend to make eating unappealing. One's meals should be attractively served and this can be a major factor in nutrition for the aged. Small tends to be more beautiful; older people need fewer calories in their diet than younger, but have similar vitamin and mineral needs. Obesity can become a real problem to the aged especially those with osteoarthritis. As the possibility of adequate exercise lessens more care should be taken to see that the diet, while being nutritious, is not weight inducing.

The changes in the digestive system are usually not as marked as those in other areas of the body. However, the decreased level of enzyme secretion and of acid in the stomach slow down the process of digestion. Large or highly seasoned meals at night may cause indigestion and flatulence which can interfere with sleep. Insomnia is frequently caused by nothing more than digestive problems and may be remedied by cutting down the fat in dairy products and other foods. Gradual loss of tone in the muscular wall of the bowel can also give rise to difficulties in defecation.

Constipation should not normally be a problem to the older person as long as there is sufficient fibre in the diet and an adequate fluid intake. Some elderly people become worried about the need for a daily bowel action, the result of incorrect stress on this as children. This is not necessary for everyone as individuals vary greatly in their needs. The habit of using aperients daily is one that should be avoided as far as possible. The addition of fresh fruit and vegetables or other fibre to the diet as well as regular exercise where possible is a far healthier and often less costly solution.

Any marked change in the normal pattern of bowel action, for example alternating constipation and diarrhoea, or unusual darkening of the stool, should be reported at once to the doctor. It can be the first indication of possible malignant disease of the colon.

The pelvic area

Changes in the bladder as ageing begins lead to a gradual reduction in its size and capacity and sometimes also a decrease in the diameter of the urethra. This alteration in capacity means that the desire to urinate may become more frequent and sometimes more urgent. Most elderly people will find that they need to go to the toilet during the night where this may not have been necessary earlier. If lighting is not adequate or there are obstacles to negotiate in getting to the bathroom this often results in falling with the possibility of a fractured bone or other injury. Nocturia may be lessened by restricting the fluid intake in the latter part of the day and by seeing that diuretics are not taken in the evening. Nervousness and anxiety can also be a cause of frequency at night and can be helped by seeing that a bottle or commode is readily accessible.

Urinary incontinence, the inability to control the bladder, is often a source of worry and loss of self-respect for the elderly person. Stress incontinence, the involuntary loss of urine when coughing, laughing, sneezing or lifting a heavy weight, often starts during the middle years and is more common in women, though it is sometimes found in men after a prostatectomy. It can be an embarrassing disorder but one which can be corrected surgically or, in milder cases, by a simple set of exercises. Kegel's exercise, as it is called, consists in alternately contracting and relaxing the pubococcygeus muscle (PCG) which forms the floor of the pelvic cavity. This can be done by the drawing up and pulling in of the muscle which normally controls urination. If this is done rhythmically ten to fifteen times several times a day muscle tone is recovered. By strengthening the PCG in this way not only can incontinence be cured or prevented but there is less likelihood of any of the pelvic organs sagging. Another bonus to the use of this exercise is that it tends to enhance vaginal and clitoral sensations in intercourse.

Incontinence may also be the result of an over-extended bladder. The desire to void is then often accompanied by an involuntary loss of urine. Again this has been the cause of many accidents among older people as they hurry to reach the bathroom in time.

It has been found useful for older people to pause when they feel the urge to rush to the toilet, wait quietly for a few seconds until the sensation of urgency passes, and then to walk calmly at a normal pace. Regular visits to the toilet after meals or hot drinks will prevent this type of incontinence and preserve peace of mind. If disposable pads are used they should be changed frequently.

Obstruction to the bladder outlet may occur as a result of narrowing of the urethra. This causes progressive frequency, urgency and nocturia because of the incomplete emptying of the bladder. This may be combined with hesitancy and intermittency and some overflow incontinence. Cystitis is likely to result from infection in the stagnant urine. Enlargement of the prostate gland in men often causes this type of obstruction. This enlargement may be quite benign or in a few cases may be caused by a malignant growth. Medical advice should always be sought in these cases.

Faecal incontinence is never a normal process of ageing and, if present, medical treatment or guidance is advised.

Sleep

Ageing may bring with it certain alterations in the patterns of sleep. Some find they apparently require fewer hours of sleep, some more, while many experience difficulty in going to sleep or wake up in the early hours of the morning. The fact that many older people may spend much of the day 'catnapping' in a chair leaves them with less need of rest and insomnia may be simply a response to this. Added activity and interest in the daytime can solve much of this frustrating wakefulness. It is wiser to avoid the use of sedation where possible and to have recourse to more natural remedies, such as daily exercise, a hot drink of milk before retiring or some herbal teas. As sleep patterns change, wakeful periods can be accepted as useful for reading, writing letters, or watching all-night television, with a cup of tea.

For some wakefulness is not a burden. As one ageing person explained: 'I enjoy being sleepless because it is then I become a mental traveller, wandering, for example, about my grandmother's house; testing my memory of its layout, wallpaper, pictures and books, especially the great folio volume of Dante's *Inferno*, whose browned and brittle leaves I used to turn over with horrified fascination, lying on the floor beside the heat-reddened coal stove.'[2] Others have found equal delight in revisiting scenes of their earlier roaming the world: 'I simply stand and gaze at the breathtaking beauty of the snow-clad alps and the deep tree-filled ravines and know that God is to be found there.'

Sleepless nights can thus become an occasion for searching for the theme of our existence, a time of looking back with wonder at the warp and woof of the tapestry of life.

♦ ♦ ♦

Chapter • 13

SOME EMOTIONAL AND MENTAL DISTURBANCES

The picture presented of the aged person serenely rocking away the last years of life is not one which is come by easily. Such peace and serenity is the outcome of a courageous and successful negotiation of many hard-won struggles on the journey. An awareness of some of the emotional changes of the later years can be helpful not only to the aged themselves but can assist those who look after them to show the understanding and concerned care often required to ease the suffering which may accompany senescence.

Emotional changes

Ageing can be a time of considerable stress and loss for many people. The changes in their society so often run counter to the values they developed throughout the years. The things they held precious, the courtesies of life, their code of ethics, no longer count for much in this new world on which they are becoming more and more dependent. The deprivation of so much — career, family, perhaps spouse or home — touches them deeply on an emotional level. Anger, frustration and depression are all as much a part of the grieving for these losses as is sadness. The altered circumstances of life may give rise to a sense of insecurity, a questioning of self-worth and an alienation from this changed society. Depleted energy levels can make it difficult for the older person to control the expression of these feelings and this is not always greeted with the tolerance and understanding it deserves.

Retirement is usually a difficult adjustment even though it may have been looked forward to for many years. To find oneself suddenly with no office to go to, no class awaiting, no job that requires doing can be a devastating experience for many. The world of work has been an inseparable part of most lives for close on half a century and the sudden cessation of involvement in it can elicit a number of emotional reactions. This is particularly the case where education for leisure has been lacking.

The sense of being lost, unneeded, insecure in a new life-style is a heavy burden to carry. The normal symptoms of crisis often accompany this change, with resultant depression and lowered self-esteem at the thought of no longer being able to contribute. A real crisis of worth may well ensue. Such was the case for Jim, a retired army colonel, who became dejected and morose when he quit the constant demands of the forces and the company of his fellow officers. On the suggestion of a friend, he found a course in household repairs, advertised in the local newspaper and in a very short time had a full-time occupation as a handyman. Calls from pensioners were answered on a voluntary basis, others paid a small fee, thus meeting the need he felt of being able to contribute to others while at the same time being involved in some culturally acceptable activity which was both useful and rewarding.

For the woman whose life-work has been in the home, it is not always easy to put up with a retired partner who has returned home to 'look for a job' and is constantly seeking some occupation in the house. Friction can result if this sudden loss of role and meaning is not properly understood.

Deprivation of the social contacts at work is also felt intensely and the retiree can become lonely, self-centred and demanding. The emotional repercussions of leaving the workforce are minimised by a 'prepared retirement' with some new occupation already planned. Then times of leisure become a source of satisfaction and enjoyment, rather than a vacuum to be filled. Several years before retirement one professional woman had already promised her future services in a legal capacity to a number of voluntary organisations.

The many losses as one ages are each a time of letting go of what is past and seeking to find new meaning in the present. The sorrow we experience when those close to us die will be accompanied by the slow process of grieving with all the emotional turmoil and pain it holds. This is a time when older people need the assurance of someone's caring presence in their lives, gently supporting and unobtrusively helping them to face the bereavement and to gradually reorganise their lives. After the death of her husband a close friend found untold support from a neighbour who simply looked in each evening to make sure that she was well. The thought of his coming helped her through the often lonely days as she knew that someone really understood her grief.

Thoughtful planning allows the older person to

remain independent and living in his or her own home for as long as possible. A variety of support systems are readily available in most areas. To become familiar with such services as meals-on-wheels, domestic assistance, transport, home-nursing and possible recreational activities even before they are required will ensure peace of mind about future needs. Some may judge it better to live in close proximity to younger family members, for example in a granny flat, or to share accommodation with a friend or relative. Again others choose to move to an independent unit in a complex for the ageing where they can remain self-reliant, have their own grounds and garden and yet feel the reassurance of help close at hand should they require it. Independent living remains preferable as long as it brings peace of mind rather than anxiety.

For the elderly, one of the hardest deprivations is their loss of independence and with it of the home that has been theirs perhaps for a life-time. The move to a hostel or home for the aged can be more traumatic than is sometimes realised and is often accompanied by severe depression and disorientation. Many older people are labelled 'confused' on their entry into institutional life, but this may be only a temporary symptom of loss. Much care and individual attention is needed in the first days of a dislocation of this kind to re-orient the person and help him or her to feel secure. Directions need to be repeated constantly at first as the disruption to an accustomed life-style can be so disturbing that new information is not easily retained. The location of toilets, times of meals and means of calling for assistance should be pointed out constantly until it is obvious that the person has regained his or her bearings. This attentive care will lessen the high degree of anxiety that invariably accompanies change. Expressions of irritability or anger or just being generally perverse may be no more than a communication of the grief that is theirs. It can be disastrous for elderly persons to be labelled as withdrawn, depressed or difficult during the first few months of such a separation. Time and understanding will help them regain their normal dispositions.

There are many reasons for the elderly to experience anxiety and fear. The welfare of children, financial difficulties, uncertainty about the future, the threat of illness, loneliness and death, can all weigh heavily on them. The thought of a loss of self-determination and of perhaps being a burden to others is a constant dread. Worse still is the possibility of becoming unable to function properly, either physically or mentally. This anxiety is understandable and can be countered by an appreciation of the concern and a gentle re-assurance from someone who really understands. Affection and the physical expression of love are a far better therapy for the anxious elder than are any drugs. For a distressed person to feel an encouraging arm around his or her shoulders brings a re-assurance words cannot.

High levels of anxiety can precipitate many physical manifestations. Palpitations, sharp chest pain, tremors, dizziness, headaches, digestive and urinary disturbances and diarrhoea can all be symptomatic of anxiety. Emotional disturbances including lack of concentration, impaired memory and a variety of phobias, such as the fear of crowds, of open spaces or of being left alone, are also common and may require psychotherapy or other professional help.

Because of the inter-relatedness of psychological and bodily factors, anxiety may reveal itself in somatic illnesses. The so-called psychosomatic diseases are very real and require treatment of the physical element as well as the psychological one. The complexity of the underlying cause often makes this type of illness more difficult to cure. Mention of this has been made in an earlier chapter on stress.

Loneliness, which is so often the fate of the old, can be one of the greatest sufferings. Close family and friends die or move away leaving an ever diminishing circle of acquaintances, few of whom can meet the need to share and reminisce together. The sense of separation inherent in loneliness is complicated by the feeling of rejection so often experienced through the loss of involvement in society. Opinions are no longer sought, the usual ways of doing things have become outmoded and there seems to be no place left for them in this modern world. There remains a deep sense of emptiness, of 'non being'. The pain of loneliness can give rise to feelings of worthlessness, alienation and self-pity or, again, can be the source of turning out in search of more satisfying relationships with others or with God. Companionship for the lonely aged, as for those at any stage of life, can save them from bitterness and cynicism and from a future which is formless, empty and without hope. But for the elderly, it can have the added advantage of a fruitful sharing with another of the riches of a lifetime. As Henri Nouwen reflected on 'the wound of loneliness' he compared it to the Grand Canyon, 'a deep incision in the surface of our existence which has become an inexhaustible source of beauty and self-understanding'.[1] It can be made this if one learns to face its pain allowing it to enhance understanding rather than doing everything possible to escape from it. As Etty Hillesum, the young Dutch Jewish woman wrote in her diary as she waited in Westerbork Barracks to be sent to her death in Auschwitz: 'With a sharp pang, all of suffering mankind's nocturnal distress and loneliness passes now through my small heart ... You know if you don't have the inner strength while you're here to understand that all the outer appearances are a passing show, as nothing beside the great splendour inside us, then things can look very black here indeed.'[2]

The losses and alienation of old age sometimes give rise to a state of depression and helplessness. This may show itself in a definable mood change with sadness, anxiety and hopelessness; or it may be masked by a smiling face and revealed by loss of appetite and weight, insomnia or simply indecisiveness. J. Grimley Evans describes atypical facial pain in women and persistent backache in men as a common symptom of masked depression. When the depression is treated the pain may persist but is no longer distressing to the patient. 'Elderly people whose depressive illnesses manifest as a persistent physical symptom may be at a particularly high risk of suicide,'[3] he warns.

The ageing who are depressed need help to find some meaning or purpose in life, even if that consists of something as small as contacting or helping at least one other person in the day. An elderly woman battling depression after her admission to a hostel was entrusted with the task of bringing another blind resident to meals and helping him cut up his food. This provided the purpose for living which she had lost on leaving her own home.

As in all cases of depression the ability to stress the good things, the gifts in life, rather than the negatives will assist the depressed person to achieve a more positive outlook. Genuine gratitude for these will promote an attitude that is other-centred and will tap into inner reserves of strength. The grateful heart soon becomes the hope-filled heart. Forms of relaxation and involvement with others, such as gardening, listening to music or playing games will encourage a turning-out from self and a more creative approach to life. If the depression is marked medication may be necessary.

Notification of a terminal illness or the awareness of some further diminishment will normally bring about emotional turmoil similar to that of the grieving process. Anger may be the first feeling registered and this can be disconcerting for friends or family in their efforts to give support. The aged person may feel lost and confused and no longer him or her true self. It may take some months before equilibrium is regained and life resumes an even tenor.

Awareness of the emotional disturbances associated with ageing can help older people to understand and be more tolerant of the changes in temperament they may be experiencing. It can also help their carers to offer the needed support, encouragement and companionship. Thus these will learn from the elderly ways in which they, in their turn, can prepare for a fruitful and serene old age.

Mental changes

Mental deterioration is frequently another cause of concern to the ageing themselves and to those who care for them. Forgetfulness, the bane of life's second half, can grow more marked in the later years. This may be the result of a decrease in the presence of chemicals needed in the transmission of messages between brain cells. In more serious cases it can indicate that a fundamental degenerative process is taking place. As Francis Braceland[4] emphasises, it is necessary to differentiate between the complaint and the performance. Those who complain most about memory loss are sometimes found to function better than those who have not registered any difficulty. Robert N. Butler, in speaking of 'benign senescent forgetfulness' points out that unless the memory loss is continuous and disabling, it is not normally a symptom of disease.

Increasing loss of memory and vagueness can be early symptoms of senile degeneration from a variety of causes including arteriosclerosis, or of Alzheimer's disease. Some of these dementias, as they are called, may arise from conditions which are curable and for this reason it is important to seek medical advice as soon as the symptoms become obvious. There is as yet no known remedy for Alzheimer's disease which, according to Dr Butler, occurs in four to six per cent of the population at present. It is a devastating condition both for the person affected and for the family members involved. Mental deterioration continues relentlessly until finally the sufferer loses touch with the world and all control over both mind and body. Death brings the only known relief. Advice as how best to care for a relative with Alzheimer's disease or any of the dementias is available from community health centres or the Alzheimer's Disease and Related Disorders Society in various parts of the world.

Confusion in the elderly can be caused by many psychological, social and physical determinants. As we have already seen grieving from loss, such as the death of a loved one or leaving a life-time home, is one of the commonest reasons and will pass in time. So also will the disorientation found in many illnesses, heart attack, pneumonia or even something as simple as a cold. Some older people become confused in social gatherings where they are suddenly surrounded by a crowd of strangers. Even changes in the accustomed furnishing of a room may well bewilder them. At times this state is recognised only by the person affected who manages successfully to hide it from others. By limiting activity or staying at home rather than risking disorientation in the larger environment, mildly confused people may succeed in living a fairly normal, if restricted, life.

Those, however, who are more markedly disoriented make this obvious to others by their inability to cope with normal living. Forgetfulness of recent happenings or of faces and names may vary in extent as people age. But loss of a sense of where they are or of time, not being able to distinguish between the days or years, are unmistakable signs of confusion. There may be difficulty in remembering how to dress or where to go for meals or which bedroom is theirs. Hard as it may be to remain patient when someone again mistakes the broom cupboard for the toilet, it helps to remember that he or she is endeavouring to remain independent and to be of help. It can be crushing to the sufferer to scold or show anger and this only adds further to the disorientation through fear of doing wrong.

Efforts to keep the elderly in touch with the reality around them are essential. Those suffering from confusion can be assisted by the constant repetition in conversation of the four main 'signposts' to prevent them losing themselves in a world of chaos: *who* they and their carers are, *when* it is, *where* they are and *what* is happening. A simple greeting such as the following can help them locate themselves and lessen anxiety: 'Andrew, I'm Jane, your wife, and it's Tuesday this morning. We're going down from the bedroom to the kitchen and I'll get your breakfast for you.' During the course of the day information can be given regularly as to the city they are in, the season of the year, the names and relationship of those they meet. Some people have found that a clock with the day, the week and the year as well as the time, is a useful aid, while others have a small board with the relevant information written where it can be constantly seen. It is important, too, to tell the confused person what you are doing, especially if you are in need of some co-operation, and to speak to him or her as to an adult not as to a child. Any instructions given will need to be very clear and to be repeated several times until they are grasped.

Hypochondriasis, another ailment in some ageing people, may be associated with anxiety or depression or may exist in a pure form. This is a neurotic disorder characterised by preoccupation with bodily functions, especially those of the gastrointestinal tract, though any system may be involved. Fear that one is inflicted with a serious disease predominates. Not infrequently an aged person with little or no outside interest develops an excessive and unhealthy concern with self, and complains of severe pain or discomfort in various parts of the body. Unlike psychosomatic disorders there is no underlying physical cause of the symptoms experienced which vary in severity. Hypochondriasis is a particularly difficult complaint to treat especially when associated with depression or high anxiety. A serious and thorough investigation is needed to convince the physician that there is no physical abnormality. This should be explained to the patient and the possible effects of emotional disturbances on the body elucidated.

Once convinced that their symptoms have been taken seriously and that there is no obvious cause apart from the anxiety or other emotional stress, many older people are willing to accept help in working to alleviate the condition. Investigation sometimes reveals a condition of constant frustration through attempting to achieve objectives which are now beyond them. Once they are reconciled to abandoning these and replacing them with realistic goals, they are able to achieve a more productive and fulfilling life. Family members or friends are also of assistance in filling in details of personality changes which have preceded the condition and in providing the encouragement to participate in rewarding occupations. A sympathetic and supportive home environment seems to be more helpful than other palliative treatment.

Paranoid changes are also found in some older people who become convinced that they are being unjustly treated, discriminated against or have become the target of other people's aggression. They tend to blame others and to become acutely sensitive and suspicious. Simple everyday events can be misinterpreted to justify their suspicions and to confirm their claims of persecution or of infidelity of a spouse. The disordered personality which shows itself in paranoid illness will be one that earlier gave evidence of extreme sensitivity and a tendency to interpret incidents falsely as being demeaning or insulting. As Braceland points out, it is rare that the normal stresses of ageing will induce such abnormal emotional or mental reactions in individuals who have shown stable personality patterns in earlier life. Those who develop any unbalanced outlook on life in their later years will usually have shown some previous difficulty in adjustment.

In fact observation shows that 'in normal men and women there is no sharp discontinuity of personality with age, but rather an increasing consistency'.[5] Characteristics of earlier life become more clearly pronounced and cherished values are more strongly held. The graciousness so often found among the very old is the outcome of a habit of politeness and consideration for others, not something acquired in later years.

Alleviation and care

The emotional problems and psychiatric disorders met with in the aged can be alleviated if those caring for them can help them to remain conscious of their dignity and worth. This is communicated in the respect demonstrated in their care or the attention to their needs. To care is to meet with patience and compassion those who are old or ill, to enter into their world bringing solace and companionship. To truly care is to stay with those who, because of brokenness of mind or body, are no longer humanly attractive or appealing, to feel with them in their isolation and loneliness, to let them know that they have value in our sight. An elderly woman, the neglected victim of Alzheimer's disease, showed a remarkable improvement when the nursing staff of the home to which she was admitted made efforts to see that she was smartly dressed, and her previous standards of grooming maintained. Though apparently completely unaware of what was happening around her, something of the consideration and respect shown her seemed to penetrate her consciousness. She lost her previous aggressiveness and appeared to be much more at peace, becoming considerably easier to tend.

In providing appropriate care for those suffering from the varying degrees of any of the dementias much can be done to ease, if not to reverse their symptoms of confusion or memory loss. They can be helped to maintain self-esteem, not to think of themselves as 'silly old people', by being encouraged to develop their full potential as far as it remains possible. This will ensure a feeling of self-worth, a lessening of loneliness and isolation, and an awareness that life can still be fun. Programmes designed to involve such people in skill development activities, social gatherings, enjoyable outings and so on, can all help to continue their involvement with others and lead to a higher quality of enjoyment of the remaining years of life. The sense of fun which had been characteristic of Vincent during his earlier life stayed with him as he underwent a degree of mental degeneration. He still brought endless pleasure to others by seeming to deliberately adopt the role of the forgetful clown in the nursing home to which he was confined.

There can be a tendency in some to address the elderly as if they were children. This is often justifiably resented, and the aged person may refuse to co-operate, feigning inability. Elders should be encouraged to remain independent for as long as feasible, to take whatever part they can in the decision making which touches them, and whenever possible to have freedom of choice rather than imposition of regulations.

Life satisfaction

Every effort should be made to ensure maximum life satisfaction for the ageing. To maintain some purpose and interest is to remain productive and emotionally stable. To keep in touch with contemporary events is to keep mentally alert and involved in society. Each has a unique contribution to make and when this is recognised and affirmed it brings with it an enthusiasm for living and a heightened self-concept.

Bernice Neugarten[6] has found that for the majority of older people there is a definite correlation between the extent of social interaction and their general psychological well-being. Some personalities, however, are able to disengage more readily and still remain highly contented and well-adjusted in life.

There is a deep need for beauty, too, in the ageing heart, as there is in all of us. So often the old can find themselves isolated amid dreary and colourless surroundings, or even in a squalor and ugliness which destroys their inner sense of worth and wholeness. Even in such situations an elderly person can do much to enliven otherwise drab surroundings. Beauty can come in many forms, perhaps in the voices and warmth of those who care for them, in a flower, a pet or in a picture to brighten bare walls. For those fortunate enough to be surrounded by nature's loveliness, a sense of hope and joy can be born from the very context of their living. For others, a flowering plant, a bird or perhaps a brightly coloured bedspread can bring something of the radiance of creation into an otherwise colourless environment. To be able to sit in the sun and feel its warmth or to spend time in a park or by the sea can all be life-giving to those who at times, however, may need the help of others to make the necessary effort to venture out of doors.

Where a number of the elderly are living together they can arrange enriching leisure occupations as a group. One Senior Citizens' Club formed a choir amongst its members and very soon they found themselves performing at social functions and travelling quite far afield to do so. Community singing can be a way of bringing people together to enjoy companionship and sharing. It may also fulfil a therapeutic function for those with memory loss, or speech difficulties resulting from a stroke, as the words of old favourites return to mind. Art, drama and the establishment of a craftshop where their handwork can be displayed for sale can all give added enthusiasm and zest for life.

Ritual, too, plays a valuable role in the lives of the aged. This may come through various celebrations, a monthly birthday party for the hostel residents involved, regular visits to the local senior citizens' club or to a care and craft group. Special feast days may be observed in religious celebrations and these extended through to the meal or other activities of the day. A communal administering of the sacrament of the sick or reconciliation brings with it a sense of being part of a pilgrim community in this latter part of life's journey.

Emotional support in these years is provided largely by the family or close friends. To keep in touch with them and to ensure that there is a warm welcome awaiting those who call may require effort but this is well worthwhile and rewarding. When writing or phoning becomes difficult it may be possible for the elderly person to seek the assistance of others in order to keep these vital relationships alive. The chance to reminisce, to recall events which have made up the pattern of the past, can help the aged to find the meaning and purpose of their existence and enables them more readily to surrender life when the moment comes.

'Wellness', an attitude which embraces the more positive approach of recognising what is right, normal and healthy in a person who may be suffering from some illness, fosters a constructive disposition in the elderly, or for that matter in persons of any age. 'I am in the best of health,' said one hospital patient who was waiting for an amputation. 'It is only just my leg that isn't well.' Wellness differs from health and can be a powerful force in the life of someone who nonetheless may be said to be chronically ill. It has been defined as 'an active process through which an individual becomes aware of and constantly makes choices towards a more meaningful existence'. To concentrate mainly on failing health or sickness is to miss the fact that in many other ways the person may be functioning in a normal healthy fashion. Wellness is concerned with the prevention of illness, with rehabilitation and with remaining as independent and as involved in decision making as possible in spite of any illness that may be present.

The elderly who have maintained an active interest and curiosity in the world around them and striven to keep mentally alert, taking part in whatever enterprises their strength permits, are most likely to enjoy a balanced and creative time of ageing. They will not find the long hours of solitude times of loneliness or tedium because they have occupations and interests to fill their minds. As an eighty-year-old once commented: 'There are so many parts of the world, so many people, so very many problems that need my prayer, I just can never get around to all of them.'

Play, too, remains as important in the later years as it is at any age. For the young it is part of their nature, for the aged its importance must often be rediscovered. The young of every species 'come into earth's system of life as if play were what they were created for. They explore, cross the normal limits of things, leap about without reason, climb too far out on limbs, and fall in the water when their curiosity fastens on something new and strange there. The young reveal the core of life's mystery: the need and opportunity for adventurous play'.[7] For the old the form of play may change but its essential purpose remains the same: to give expression to the creativity, freedom and capacity to wonder and to dream which is theirs by right. To play, to fantasise and use imagination are all key powers within the human person. They lead to daring exploration of the possible and above all to the ability to laugh, that most healing process for the human spirit. To play with words in humour is to unfold a gentle wit, the precursor and companion of true wisdom.

♦ ♦ ♦

Chapter • 14

SUFFERING AND DEATH

A young man struck down by a terminal illness in his twenties once wrote: 'I had struggled for months to accept this call to give up life before it had fully begun for me, to lie here in pain able to do nothing, when there is so much I want to do and to be. Then one night as I was trying to pray and finding only darkness, I suddenly saw that this is my work, the vocation I'm called to: to make my home in suffering while I live, to let it do its work in me and through me maybe reach out in some way to others. The fight to accept this illness has now ended as I know the purpose of my life. The pain is still there but now it has its meaning. Instead of speaking to me of inability to do the things I want to, it has become the mission of these last few months of life.'

The struggle for most, the fear that overwhelms them, is not so much the death they know must be faced but the diminishment which may lie before them and the suffering it may well entail. This is what nature rebels against; it is this that is so dreaded. The mystery of the need for pain and suffering in this world, and it is mystery, is something we cannot fathom and cannot adequately explain.

Suffering

Suffering has been part of history as far back in time as we can travel, and has defied all attempts to understand its *raison d'être* on a purely intellectual level. There seems no way of escaping or avoiding it, no cure that frees us from its consequences. The writers of one after another of the books of the bible wrestle with the problem of suffering in the persons of original man and woman, of Job, of Jeremiah and of the suffering Servant of Israel. Perhaps of all their writings the Book of Job presents the most graphic picture of a human touched for no apparent reason by baffling loss, destruction and physical torment. Its writer elaborates his own efforts to come to an understanding of something that seemed so meaningless, and undeserved. Why should such a series of tragedies occur? The response was not an answer but a revelation of the greatness of the creator — 'God is supreme' — (Job 36:22) and a recognition, on Job's part, that God is all powerful: '... what you conceive you can perform.' (Job 42:2) Here was a willingness to place trust where trust was most deserved.

More modern writers have filled libraries with their treatises as to why suffering is part of the human condition and have found no satisfactory explanation — for its presence remains mystery. The one answer, which keeps echoing in reply to our bewilderment as to its place in a universe created by a loving God, comes to us in the words of the prophet Isaiah: 'My ways are not your ways ... Yes, the heavens are as high above earth as my ways are above your ways, my thoughts above your thoughts.' (Isaiah 55:8-9) And like Job we acknowledge that we cannot call God to account, but that his wisdom may give meaning to what seems meaningless to us.

We can only ask why, and as Rainer Maria Rilke, who himself suffered greatly as a child, warns us: 'Do not now seek the answers, which cannot be given you because you would not be able to live them ... Live the questions now. Perhaps you will then gradually, without noticing it, live along some distant day into the answer.'[1] We may then perhaps discover that the real answer is not an explanation, but a presence, that of God himself. The mystery of human suffering may prove, finally, to be the mystery of our transformation.

Suffering then is part of our being human and remains an enigma. We can only ask the question 'why' and in the asking recognise that it may be the wrong question. The 'why' is less important than the 'how'. How do we approach the mystery of suffering, how do we accept and cope with pain when it comes? The answer to that question will reveal itself only when we meet suffering ourselves. It will depend on what we discover to be its meaning for us and on the strength that will be given to endure it. For unless we find some meaning in it, it will become intolerable, leading to bitterness and despair.

Victor Frankl discovered in the midst of the cruelty and debasement of a concentration camp that transcendent love, *agape*, was a possibility for the human person. It is he who quotes Nietzsche as saying: 'He who has a "why" to live can bear with almost any "how".'[2] It was Frankl who gave substance to these words. He could endure what brought millions of others to their death because he knew what it meant to love his torturers with selfless love. Indeed, almost any trial can be born once we know that it has a meaning.

Dorothy Soëlle, the German theologian, suggests that the most important question we can ask about suffering is not what is its cause, but whom does it serve? Is the outcome of the anguish born by so many directed towards good, towards God, or towards the evil powers? Of itself suffering has no intrinsic value. To embrace it for itself is morbid, even masochistic. The value, if there is to be any, comes from our response to it. It is we who can give pain a positive or a negative meaning in our lives; can let it transform us or let it fill us with resentment and self-seeking. The more important question then is not from where does it come, what is the reason for suffering; but rather to where is it leading, what will be its outcome in my life?

How then can pain transform us? What could be its purpose in our lives?

There is a mysterious power in suffering to open up unexplored spaces in the human spirit, to reveal new capacities, and fresh areas of sensitivity. Pain is known to break open undiscovered powers of creativity or genius. Terminal cancer led one young man to give expression to his pain and loss, for the first time, in a book of poems, published only after he had died. Musicians still marvel at the beauty and sensitivity of Beethoven's string quartets written in the years of his greatest pain and anguish. The last self-portrait of Rembrandt depicts the haggard, pain-filled face of a man broken by suffering and yet its execution reveals a strength of expression and genius not evident before.

Pain calls forth the best, or worst, in the human personality. It enables us to go beyond ourselves to a self-transcendence which leads to a deep concern for others, an ability to feel with them in their anguish. We cannot be truly compassionate or meet another deeply in their pain unless we have ourselves experienced something similar. Suffering creates an openness to receive others in distress and perhaps bring healing to them because they are understood; we have been there too. 'That deep shade of compassion and love which is born in us is like no other,' a friend who suffered from recurrent depression wrote to his fellow sufferers. 'It is born in anguish and terror, forged in the fires of loneliness, and given depth by the love of God. At our weakest moment a strength is born. We have learnt to look at and love our fellow man, in a manner that no one else will know. We will never be the same again.'[3]

Compassion, the ability to welcome and to feel with others, is true hospitality and is born within the heart which has been laid open by pain. The invitation in the gospel to be 'perfect just as your heavenly Father is perfect', (Matthew 5:48) speaks, according to scripture scholars, of the call to be compassionate just as the heavenly Father is compassionate. For Meister Eckhart, a fifteenth century mystic, the best name known for God was Compassion. The extent of that compassion has been revealed in Jesus whose heart was deeply moved on seeing the crowds, the sick, the poor and the hungry, who wept on hearing of a close friend's death. His was a gut reaction, an anguish from the depth of his being. He was poor with the poorest, sick with the sick, hungry with those without food. It is this compassion, an enduring with the other, that we are invited to share. It is only when pain has touched us personally that we are truly qualified to show this deep concern for others, to enter into their vulnerability and their powerlessness.

A beautiful and moving example of this self-transcendence and solicitude for others was found in the concentration camp of Ravensbruck. When the liberating troops entered the camp they found a torn scrap of paper beside a dead child. On it was written this prayer:

> *O Lord, remember not only the men and women of good will, but also those of ill will. But do not remember all the suffering they have inflicted on us; remember the fruits we have bought, thanks to this suffering — our comradeship, our loyalty, our humility, our courage, our generosity, the greatness of heart which has grown out of all this, and when they come to judgement, let all the fruits which we have borne to be their forgiveness.*[4]

'All I know,' wrote Pierre d'Harcourt reflecting on his own experience in a similar camp, 'is that when it became hardest of all for men to behave like decent human beings, they spread their wings and rose to great heights; and when the strains and temptations were removed, they sank into the mud.'[5]

This rising to the heights is the opening up of our real greatness and suffering has the power to bring to birth the true and best in each one and to attune both mind and heart more finely. There are elements in all of us that come into existence only when suffering touches them and calls them forth. The little child in the cancer ward found what was in him to become when his own understanding of pain prompted him to give his bear, the one support he had, to the boy in the bed next to his. 'Because,' he said, 'if you hold him tight, he'll get you through the worst times.'

Suffering, too, opens up not only the power of giving but also the ability to receive. This receptivity takes place in the centre of one's being, the self. And the greatest gift we are able to receive within the self is that of God's life-giving presence. Pain, in some strange way, seems to have the power to remove the obstacles to receiving this, even though we may not be aware of it. Often when God seems furthest from us, he is closest. 'Once the human life is broken,' Rumi, the Sufi mystic explains 'the God-wave can enter in.' When the retaining wall holding back the ocean crumbles, the tranquil waters of the harbour become turbulent and stormy, but at the same time filled with a vigour and vitality not there before. Once this happens in life we are brought to understand with Teilhard de Chardin that 'God must, in some way or other, make room for himself, hollowing us out and emptying us, if he is finally to penetrate into us'[6] and take possession of us. It is pain that empties us, if only we allow it, for his filling.

One of the most distressing trials towards the end of life can be the darkness which comes upon so many; a darkness of loss, of bewilderment, sometimes of rejection and of the sense of uselessness and failure. T.S. Eliot describes such a condition in the *Four Quartets* when he writes in 'East Coker':

> *O dark, dark, dark. They all go*
> *into the dark ...*
> *I said to my soul, be still,*
> *and let the dark come upon you*
> *which shall be the darkness of*
> *God ...*

I said to my soul, be still, and
wait without hope
For hope would be hope for the
wrong thing;
Wait without love, for love would
be love of the wrong thing;
There is yet faith;
But the faith and the love and the
hope are all in the waiting ...
So the darkness shall be the light
and the stillness, the dancing.

There is something mysterious about the dark and God's action in it which cannot be seen but can only be guessed. Our origins have been in darkness and in darkness we lived the first nine months of existence. There will be recurrences of that darkness, the creative darkness of God, during the course of life's journey. These will appear at times as an aching void, at times as an arid wasteland, but they will always be occasions of potential transformation and more abundant growth. The deepest pain of all may not be that which comes from without, but that centred in our inmost being.

There are, all around, people whose very presence can draw us into the mystery of God's action in the darkness of human suffering: those who are battling with the blackness of depression or struggling to endure physical pain; those lost in the wilderness of confusion; some grieving the death of loved ones; others called to let go of health or faculties, of home or relatives. We can only wonder at the extent of human suffering and believe that the answer to it all may lie in the ongoing creation of the human spirit.

'Pain is not simply a puzzle, an enigma; it is a kerygma, an announcement.'[7] C.S. Lewis speaks of pain as 'God's megaphone to rouse a deaf world'.[8] It is a constant reminder of mortality, of the seriousness of life, and the closeness of death. It can lead to a realisation of the depths and heights the human person is capable of reaching. It strengthens character and enlarges the capacity to give.

But perhaps above all it is a call to remind us that we are living a mystery, commissioned in some way to 'make up all that is still to be undergone by Christ for the sake of his Body, the Church'. (Corinthians 1:24) As members of his Body, we carry into the twentieth century the continuation of the redemption wrought on Calvary. This does not mean that the redemption achieved there was incomplete, but rather in the words of John Paul II: 'It seems to be part of the very essence of Christ's redemptive suffering that this suffering requires to be unceasingly completed ... [remaining] ... always open to all love expressed in human suffering.'[9] Every human anguish, lovingly accepted, thus 'completes the suffering of Christ just as the Church completes his redemptive work'.[10] In union with Christ who continues his Paschal Mystery in this world, we are called through suffering to a shared experience with him not only of the cross, but also of his resurrection. Teilhard de Chardin speaks of this communion as the Christification of human suffering. It is the part each one can play in bringing life to the world, and salvation and enrichment to others.

The call then is not only to accept our life as we age but also our diminishments and sufferings. We are challenged not only to accept, but even to love, the pain that comes with ageing, not to enjoy or take pleasure in it, but to love it for its meaning in our lives and in the lives of those whom we can reach through it. Martin Israel writes with profound insight:

'This is the end of personal suffering — to prove oneself worthy of it. For it is the supreme fulfilment of becoming fully human — and, therefore, starting to partake fully of the divine nature to which we were called at the moment of our creation.'[11]

Perhaps the answer to all our questioning about the mystery of human pain can be found in the discovery of the Little Prince: '"What makes the desert beautiful is that somewhere it hides a well"...' And de Saint Exupéry writes: 'And, as I walked on so, I found the well, at daybreak.'[12]

Death

In *Children's Letters to God* there is one contribution which expresses much of what is in the depths of each one's heart. A little child writes:

> Dear God,
> What is it like when you die? Nobody will tell me. I just want to know. I don't want to do it.
>
> Your friend,
> Mike

We would all like to put that question to God, especially those who know they are approaching the end of life's journey. Yet, on the whole we seem reluctant even to ask it of each other. Once, as I was speaking on ageing to a group of elderly sisters in Ireland, an eighty-three-year-old tentatively enquired: 'Why is it we never talk together about dying?' It seemed strange to her that here in a home for the ageing, no one ever raised in public the most important issue for them all.

Death for some is an event to be welcomed, a celebration to be shared amongst friends. A few years ago, a friend, when told that she was dying, invited those closest to her to celebrate this entry into eternal life while she and they could still enjoy this good news together. She wanted to commemorate life and all that it had held for her while welcoming the new life that lay ahead. So she held a party.

But for others there is a deep fear of death. Its announcement is often greeted with denial. Jack Dominian noted that those of his clients who were preoccupied with the apprehension of death were those who lacked a clear sense of their identity together with a marked insecurity and lack of self-acceptance. The dread of losing the customary support of family or friends and confronting the unknown that lay ahead was too much for them to face. Their anxiety showed itself in a fear of complete disintegration: 'Nothing will be left of me.' To help overcome such an attitude is often the task of those who care for the ageing and those approaching death. A sense of identity and self-worth can be communicated by the care, respect and affection shown them and the patience with which we listen to their fears. 'I never knew I mattered to anyone before I came here,' one resident of a nursing home confided, 'and now I feel I'm someone.'

'There is a season for everything ... a time for giving birth, a time for dying.' (Ecclesiastes 3:1) When Paul speaks to the Corinthians of his own diminishment and his approaching death, he tells them: 'Though this outer man of ours may be falling into decay, the inner man is renewed day by day.' (2 Corinthians 4:16) In the Hebrew mind there was no split between body and spirit but only a unity of personhood. The outer man Paul speaks of, then, is the whole person as susceptible to the pressures, concerns and sufferings of this world, subject to the power of dissolution and decay. The inner man is the one whose spiritual growth progresses even as his bodily strength and powers decline and who will know full life only in the age to come. The former experiences corruptibility, the latter is imperishable.

These two aspects of diminishment and movement to final fulfilment, full personhood, go on concurrently. Life is a constant series of little deaths, times of letting go, of the renunciation of power and in the end even of space. We move from the wide expanse of an active involvement in the world, to the limited space and occupation of home and garden, then of room, until finally we are restricted to the narrow confines of a bed. Each of these small dyings, these crises, can help break through to the deeper meaning of our lives thus strengthening the inner person. In each we can open spaces in our being to receive God and the new life which is his gift.

It is surely not simply a coincidence that since the carnage of World War II, the horror of Hiroshima and the slow death of millions in the concentration camps of Europe, theologians have turned their attention more and more to a theology of death, seeking a deeper understanding of its mystery. Rahner, and with him many others, have tried to fathom further the transformation which meets us in our dying. He maintains that death does not come as something thrust upon us and in which we take no part. He sees death as an act one personally performs. This is not to say that we choose the time and place, for the Son of Man will come like a thief in the night 'at an hour you do not expect'. (Matthew 24:44) It does mean that we take an active role, adopt an attitude and make a free choice for or against God in our dying.

Death marks the beginning of the final and definitive state in the life to come. But this is not something determined only in our concluding moments. We become what we have chosen to be, what we have gradually made ourselves by the free and deliberate decisions of a lifetime. If life has been directed towards the service and love of God and of our fellow human beings, it is this love which will blossom out spontaneously and choose communion when this is offered finally. If, however, it has remained ego-centred, proud and self-sufficient, the roots of selfishness, unless cut across before that last moment of decision, will lead inevitably to a deliberate choice of separation and isolation for all eternity.

At the moment of death, then, two things are happening: the natural separation, which we in the West speak of as the separation of the spiritual principle of life, the soul, from the body, and also the spiritual achievement of full life. The former comes from without, the latter is an activity from within, an act we personally perform.

Let us look then at what Rahner hypothesises as the result of this change in our existence. During life's course it is through the body that we see and touch and enjoy the universe about us. Our relationship to other people, to nature and to the world is mediated through our body. When, in death, the soul ceases to be united to the body, it ceases, too, to give it its distinct entity and lets it go its own way to corruption and decay. This is no more than a continuation of what has been happening in a lesser way throughout our lifetime. From the moment of birth as we struggle to master the environment, the world begins to erode our energies, our biological powers and even our bodily form. As our body gradually diminishes the first effects are felt of that separation which will result in its final disintegration.

The human soul which lives on is, however, destined by its very nature to be linked with matter. During life this connection has been through the body, which is but one part of the whole material world. Once separated from the body at death, the soul opens itself in an unmediated way to all matter: in Rahner's words it becomes 'all-cosmic'. It does not enter some non-worldly sphere but remains related to the world, so intimately connected with the depths of the cosmos that 'it can now exercise a direct influence on material reality and on the personal, spiritual being of men and women who are so closely connected with the cosmos'.[13] This does not mean that the soul becomes omnipresent but rather that it becomes a 'co-determining factor in the universe, so far as the latter is the ground of the personal life of other spiritual-corporeal beings'.[14]

Death opens us, therefore, to a new and closer relationship not only to the world but to all those who are still living in it. To those who grieve the loss of a loved one, it is comforting and strengthening to know that they are not cut off from those they love but can be even more intimately united to them. Though different, in that the body no longer speaks of presence, their relationship can be even closer than before.

It is only in death that we can come to a complete sense of who we are, for in life the mind is darkened by the functioning of the body. Once it leaves the body, the soul, the person, is free to fulfil wholly its proper activities. It can fully grasp the depths of its own being and its relationship to the universe. The natural separation which occurs at death leads to a loss of our spiritual-corporeal nature only to initiate, according to Rahner, a spiritual-cosmic relationship.

A personal fulfilment which is both final and definitive occurs at the same instant. We surrender life as we have known it through the years only to have hands free to accept a fullness of life undreamt of earlier. We become the person we have slowly fashioned through the decisions of a life-time. These have mapped and shaped our journey and determine who we ultimately become.

Death need not take us by surprise. The whole of life is filled with opportunities to rehearse this final passage. The ready letting go of youth, of health, of plans and perhaps of friends, when this is asked of us, can all become a preparation for the last great renunciation that each is called upon to make. To 'befriend' death through taking time to ponder on the richness of its meaning will help us come to peace with the thought of dying. It is a step each one must take alone. No one else can share it as they may have shared our living. But when we take time to recall how surely God has held us through the many little deaths of life any fear should be allayed. We know that he will sustain us just as surely in that last moment of demise.

Nonetheless when the tidings of approaching death reach us, it will be normal to react just as we have done when confronted with any of life's crises. Dr Elizabeth Kübler-Ross, the person who is probably most responsible in our day for permitting death to become again a topic to be aired more openly, describes the five major steps normally passed through before one comes to terms with dying. These constitute the typical grieving process when death approaches or when we mourn the loss of someone dear to us.

She identifies first a time of *denial* which so often follows the initial shock: 'It can't be true . . . not me.' Until one has the ability to cope with a situation, he or she does not take in its reality. This is a natural psychological defence. It is only when the person has the strength and readiness to deal with the thought of impending death that it will gradually be let in to consciousness. A terminally ill patient who is gently prepared can hear and accept such news more readily than one who is told abruptly or without true sensitivity.

Denial will normally continue until the person is ready to accept the news. It may take many different forms. Some refuse to accept the medical evidence and go from one doctor to another seeking a different diagnosis: some continue planning into the future as if nothing had occurred; others just refuse to hear. Those close to the failing person are often only too willing to support and maintain this stage of denial, not realising that the grieving process then is hindered and acceptance of the reality of dying is delayed. To remain in this state of denial does not help the person in any way.

The second stage, that of *anger*, is one during which there is a turmoil of emotions, of irritability, fear, impatience or of becoming demanding, envious of those in better health, and often very angry. Feelings of rage, resentment and envy break to the surface once denial has ended. This is a normal aspect of the grief process but one which can be distressing for both patient and relatives, and often tends to alienate those who could be most helpful. One daughter felt she could no longer visit her dying father because of his anger. She did not realise that this had little or nothing to do with her and that what her father needed most was someone to whom he could safely give expression to his feelings.

In time this may be replaced by a time of *bargaining*, and perhaps regrets, of praying to be able to do 'just this before I die', perhaps 'to see my daughter married, my son graduate'. This can also be an occasion of looking back, of self-reproach or guilt: '... if only I had acted differently, had taken care, or had not invited my friend on that excursion in the first place.'

As the realisation of the real consequences of the condition deepens there comes a feeling of isolation, loss, depression and despair. This is probably the hardest part of the grieving process for most, a time of feeling cut off, not understood, and profoundly alone. Dr Kübler Ross points out that a dying patient may experience two types of *depression*, one arising from the loss of so much through their illness, the other in preparation for the final separation from this world. The former may be eased by reassurance that all is well at home, that children and loved ones are happy and secure. The latter is best helped not by encouragements and looking towards the positives of life, but rather by giving the patient the opportunity to express his or her grief and sorrow for the impending loss of all that has been precious. This is often done best in a silent communication of the depth of one's caring, perhaps by touch, a stroking of the hair, a holding of the hand or by simply being with the other in his or her pain.

If a terminally ill person has been able to work through these stages of grieving then *acceptance* of death will come naturally as the final step. With this there is a sense of peace and of silent waiting, not necessarily of happiness but just of acceptance of what has become inevitable. Not all reach this stage of final acceptance partly because their grieving process has in some way been blocked. They may die in anger or in deep depression which makes their passing all the more filled with sorrow for those who love them.

These five steps are not always clearly defined and there may be a certain degree of fluctuation back and forth between the stages, especially that of depression. In the same way grieving after the loss of someone dear to us may go through a process which is not always easy to recognise. At times the bereaved person does not reach acceptance but continues to live on in a state of permanent depression. To allow and even assist patients to move through these stages of grieving does not mean that we or they give up the fight for life or the hope of a cure. It is this hope which so often helps them through their times of pain or loneliness.

Some people approaching death need help not only to move through the grieving process but also to come to the point of being able to surrender life. An opportunity to share their feelings of anxiety and fear of the unknown with someone who has the time to really listen while they talk may free some sufficiently to enable them to let go. Sometimes an unspoken desire can be intuited and satisfied, or help given to forgive a hurt or rejection. Only then do they feel ready to release their hold on life. It frequently happens that the dying person will hold fast to life until a special occasion, a child's birthday or Christmas Day, has passed. Others may be waiting to say goodbye to a family member or a loved companion. At times the need is to have someone pray with them a special prayer or simply to communicate the courage they need by a hand clasp or by being present quietly at the bedside. This can give the strength required to choose death.

One thirteen-year-old boy expressed his need and that of many others in a letter written to the doctors and nurses in the hospital where he was dying of leukaemia:

I am dying ...
... No one likes to talk about
such things. In fact, no one likes
to talk about much at all ...
I am the one who is dying. I
know you feel insecure, don't
know what to say, don't know
what to do. But please believe me,
if you care, you can't go wrong.
Just admit that you care. This is
what we search for.
We may ask for whys and
wherefores, but we really don't
want answers.
Don't run away. Wait. All I want
to know is that there will be
someone to hold my hand when I
need it.
I'm afraid ...
I've never died before ...

The mystery of death is the obscurity of the unknown. We may see others die, may hear reports of peace and joy from those who have had near-death experiences, may know well what theologians teach, but we have not yet experienced death and so it remains a deep mystery and for some a source of anxiety and fear. In blind faith we can only hold to the words of Jesus, 'I am going now to prepare a place for you ...' (John 14:2), and know that if our dying is in communion with his so shall our rising be. We, too, shall share in a boundless joy eternally bestowed. Death then becomes truly the doorway to life and the sacrament of our fulfilment.

♦ ♦ ♦

Chapter • 15

A SPIRITUALITY OF THE LATER YEARS

Teilhard de Chardin has captured something of the very essence of our intimacy with God during the later years of life as he prayed: 'It was a joy to me, O God, in the midst of the struggle, to feel that in developing myself I was increasing the hold you have upon me; it was a joy to me, too, under the inward thrust of life or amid the favourable play of events, to abandon myself to your providence. Now that I have found the joy of utilising all forms of growth to make you, or let you, grow in me, grant that I may willingly consent to this last phase of communion in the course of which I shall possess you by diminishing in you.'[1]

If, as we have seen, a spirituality consists of the response of the whole person to God, that response must come from the depth of one's being, from one's unique humanness, which is moving to integrity and wholeness, even while the body may be diminishing. The spiritual is not limited to a single area of life but embraces the whole of existence. It is the ground of our desires, questionings and fears; the basis of our friendships and self-searching; the source of creativity and the discovery of new talents. It welcomes continued growth as well as the signs of diminishment. It is through the loving acceptance of this final depletion that ultimate communion with God will be achieved.

'Grant,' Teilhard continues, 'that I may recognise you under the species of each alien and hostile force that seems bent upon destroying or uprooting me. When the signs of age begin to mark my body, and still more when they touch my mind; when the ill that is to diminish me or carry me off strikes from without or is born within me; when the painful moment comes in which I suddenly awaken to the fact that I am ill or growing old; and above all that last moment when I feel I am losing hold of myself and am absolutely passive within the hands of the great unknown forces that have formed me; in all those dark moments, O God, grant that I may understand that it is you ... who are painfully parting the fibres of my being in order to penetrate into the very marrow of my substance and bear me away within yourself.'

These 'dark moments' of which he speaks, these deprivations, are not confined to those which touch the body. God's coming to invade our lives may be through the loss of role, of status, power and influence, even of home and cherished friends, sometimes through financial hardship or through isolating loneliness. All these are part of the emptying by which we are opened to the transforming action of God. We are reminded of the 'kenosis' of Jesus of which Paul speaks: 'He did not cling to his equality with God, but emptied himself ... and being as all men are, he was humbler yet, even to accepting death, death on a cross.' (Philippians 2:6–8) Only in this way could he be instrumental in accomplishing his Father's plan.

It is in this emptiness that we come to a sense of our poverty of heart. We cannot of ourselves reach God, but must turn to him in hope knowing that it is the heart he sees and its desires, not the accumulation of good works. It is for him to fill the void within us, to satisfy our longings. In time we learn to let go of our own creations and be content with the person he created us to be.

Life's evening heralds for many the advent of darkness. 'The dark night of the elderly' can be a time of rootlessness, confusion and a touching of rock bottom. God's absence is more apparent than his presence and prayer seems sterile and monotonous. The sense of uselessness which haunts the aged can be a reminder that true value lies not in *what* is done but in *who* they are. It is for them to bear witness to the beauty and satisfaction of being a person of God, the one he wished for in the first place.

I once watched a gifted teacher of small children explain to a group of four- and five-year-olds the purpose of their creation. As they sat wide-eyed and expectant, she drew from a container a series of pottery vessels, a cup, a jug, a teapot and so on. Each was recognised and named. For it was the name that showed the purpose for which the thing was made. Then as she held up a teapot and suggested she might use it to eat her breakfast from, there were shouts of protest. Surely a teapot was for making tea and the bowl was fitting for breakfast. To use either differently would make it lose its value. The potter had given each a name and this clearly showed his reason for fashioning it. They, too, had been given a name and with it a special place in God's creation. The divine Potter who had crafted them wanted each one for a very special purpose which no one else could possibly fulfil. Eyes shone and faces lit up as these tiny children saw clearly the importance of their place in the plan of the universe. No point to want to be a jug if God had created you a mug — he didn't need another jug.

How often we wish that we could in some way be other than we are. The acceptance of our unique reality is critical to our relationship with the God who moulded, formed and named each one. It is in the uniqueness of this being that we find our place in the pattern of creation. To wish to be otherwise would be to seek a different place in the cosmic whole already planned. The meaningfulness of life lies in this singular destiny envisaged for each one from all eternity. 'One's own limited and often apparently fruitless efforts gain potency when understood as part of God's universal plan.'[2] It is in the final emptying, hollowing out and darkness that God himself completes the work of transformation, catching up our paltry efforts into the history of redemption. His love for his creation is unconditional, does not depend on its failures or successes. It is the preciousness of our being that allures him, not the extent of our activity or giftedness.

It is not that God condones our faults or ignores our brokenness. Just as the potter rethrows the uncentred clay or mends the shattered vessels, his mercy awaits recognition of the areas of our life which are still in need of healing. Only then can he restore the original integrity. Late adulthood can be a time of reconciliation. When speaking of mid-life we appreciated the importance of healing as memories surfaced from the past and old wounds began to be refelt. This becomes even more imperative as life approaches its end. One of the important tasks now is to review the whole of life, looking back at times both good and bad, seeking healing and forgiveness for the injuries of the past, and searching there for the motif which has inspired our intimacy with God.

In relaxed moments of prayer memories often emerge bringing with them the pain of forgotten hurts or set-backs, or the sense of failure or regret. It is these feelings that are the place of a healing which can happen only if they are allowed fully into consciousness. To convey pain, disappointment or bitterness to the Lord and to allow the touch that cured the leper to heal it, too, is often to see new meaning in what has happened in the past. The good that has sprung from an apparent evil may alter one's perception. An employee of a large firm found that the unjust dismissal from a clerical job resulted in his learning other skills and discovering that he had a talent for building and renovating houses. The indignation which had weighed on him for many years changed, in the moment of healing, to a sense of gratitude that his life had followed the pattern that it had.

Forgiveness, which is an essential part of healing, may not be easy to attain. It is important then to realise that it lies in the will rather than in the feelings. If, indeed, one can truly want to pardon and wish another well, then forgiveness of the person is there, though condemnation of the action must remain.

It can be even more difficult at times to pardon oneself. As Jung points out: 'That I forgive an insult, that I love my enemy in the name of Christ — all these are undoubtedly great virtues ... But what if I should discover ... the most impudent of all offenders, the very enemy himself — these are within me and that I stand in need of the alms of my own kindness — that I myself am the enemy who must be loved — what then?'[3] Do we not then so often condemn and harshly treat ourselves? To be open to the forgiveness and healing of God is to be able also to pardon ourselves, and to be gentle and compassionate to the adversary within.

Memories of the past which have undermined growth can in this way be turned into rich material for future harvesting. Recalling, too, the pleasant occasions of life can bring a sense of well-being, peace and satisfaction. In later years, when self-esteem can so easily be threatened, heart and strength can be gained from recalling earlier enjoyment and times when expressions of respect and love were given us. We feel the stronger, too, for appreciating the many different ways in which we have contributed.

Reviewing life in this way initiates a host of reminiscences. The telling and re-telling of their story must be respected in the aged for this is the way in which they come to a possession of themselves. As one author claims: 'the only way to capture a self extended over time is through story.'[4] This telling of one's story creates a capacity to take hold of all of life. Only then, when faced with death, can one surrender it freely, with composure and serenity.

Looking back at the journey taken becomes a prayer, the prayer of reminiscence. It will surely give rise to times of puzzlement, of regret and often of compunction. The story of two men in their disappointment and confusion can bring enlightenment and strength to those who cannot understand much of what has happened on the road of life. If only things had worked out otherwise, the disciples would not have had to flee the city and make this journey to the village of Emmaus. The countryside around was green with the new growth which comes with spring, but their hearts were winter-like within them. All their hopes were dashed by the happenings of these last days. The one in whom they put their trust had indeed failed in what he had set out to do. What hope was left?

It was only when they allowed a stranger into their conversation that he could show them that what appeared as failure was indeed success. Was it not this that Jesus had in reality come to do? Gradually their hearts began to burn within them as they finally glimpsed the meaning of it all.

The aged, too, need to invite Jesus into this 're-collection' of the past. It is he who will open up the scripture of their lives, will throw light into the dark recesses of the past, will show the gains which first appeared as losses. Gathered in this way these fragments begin to fit together as a whole. What may at first have seemed contradiction begins to make some sense. Then it is discovered that true beauty lies, not in the absence of the ugly, but in the proper blending of the two, just as in the midst of nature's greatest grandeur lies hidden the dark, dank, rotting vegetation which nourishes the tall trees. The dark, hidden failures and disappointments keep us rooted in a humble acknowledgement of our dependence on God's mercy and the truth that we, too, are 'as all men [and women] are.' (Philippians 2:7) This brings us 'to recognise, even celebrate, a deeper truth — that no one "earns" his way, that life's meaning is more a gift than a reward.'[5]

Remembering the past in this way leads also to a deepening of self-knowledge. A meditative reflection on former events discloses much about the identity of the self which is expressed within them. 'There is great need, as one comes to the closing part of life, to find the shape, not of the things we did so much as the self who did them in the midst of rapid change and discontinuity.'[6] As we touch this profoundest level of being, we learn to recognise the unfolding of the God-life within and our co-creative role in the world that lies about us.

We cannot but affect the world in which we live, either by bringing new life and hope to it or by hindering growth. Each person whose life we touch is in some way altered by this contact. Even the universe exults in its celebration, for it is, in itself, 'a great celebration of that ultimate mystery whence it came'.[7] Joy promotes joy, sadness gloom, and bitterness discontent. The aged can be bringers of hope, of inspiration and new strivings. By a simple word of love and affirmation, new possibilities can come to birth in others. One very old friend became such a source of growth for a group of young students who called in regularly 'to visit', but in reality to receive from her a word of appreciation and praise or simply a smile that told them they were loved.

For love is the great gift the elderly have to bring to an alienated and strife-torn world. Tested and refined by the vicissitudes of a life-time it becomes in the mature adult a detached and nonpossessive affection for the other, a love that is ready to give selflessly in service and to enter with compassion into the sufferings of others. The aged have learnt that paradoxically it is in giving that one receives, and in selflessness that one becomes more integrally one's true self.

Prayer can become simpler for the elderly, perhaps because they are more at home with God. This does not imply in any way that it is easier. The darkness which so often accompanies these years can lead into a wilderness where there seem to be no paths and no direction. A sense of hopelessness may be overwhelming, an increasing feeling of the uselessness of it all. And yet even the birdsongs, the colour of flowers and sea and the glory of the stars at night are all useless in this way. It is in this uselessness, this inability to *do* anything, that is discovered the value of *being* the person God created us to be. The whole of life becomes a prayer, of opening up to the reality of who we are in our relationship to God.

It is enough now to be receptive, open to a world suffused with beauty, to the warmth of friendship, the joy of being needed, even the pain of misunderstanding or of loss. It is in all these ways that we are receptive, too, to the God who comes through his creation, his word in scripture or in the silent depths of our inner being. Younger people are often preoccupied with their side of prayer, but with age the realisation comes that it is God's side which really matters. To be open to receive love is a greater gift by far than striving to express it. A beautiful depiction of this truth is found engraved on a Hebridean altar: 'I am serene because I know Thou lovest me. Because Thou lovest me, nothing can wreathe me from my peace. Because Thou lovest me I am as one to whom all good has come.'

A form of prayer which many find helpful at this time of life is what is sometimes called the prayer of the heart or centring prayer. This has been described by the author of the *Cloud of Unknowing* as entering into 'the darkness of unknowing that lies between you and your God'.[8] This movement into the inner depths in imageless contemplation brings an awareness that 'at the very root of our being we are in constant, immediate and inescapable contact with the infinite power of God'.[9]

To pray the prayer of the heart requires a certain relaxation and a posture which is comfortable while at the same time, conducive to remaining alert. With all preoccupations and concerns relinquished and mind disengaged one can more readily enter the deepest place of the spirit, the centre that is the self. Prayer then consists of just *being*, in faith and love, in the presence of the invisible God who has made his home in this centre. To help reach and stay in this place a meaningful word or phrase may well be used occasionally. This maintains and speaks of presence, just as a word whispered now and then to a friend tells of love. It can also gently draw one back to the centre when attention wanders. At the end of such a time an unhurried repetition of some or all of the phrases of the Our Father, letting their meaning gradually unfold, will be a gentle transition to the world of everyday concerns.

One religious sister wrote of her experience of this form of prayer: 'It seemed to me that I moved to a new home in the Cloud of Unknowing ... A house gift, on the occasion of my moving in, was the instantaneous disappearance of loneliness as the characteristic tonality of my life from early childhood. Within the Cloud, I now felt at ease, not like a gauche and unwelcome guest, but like a loved member of the family.'[10]

Loneliness when touched by God's presence becomes a place of solitude where we can seek 'the face of the invisible who cannot be found unless we become lost in him, who is invisible.'[11] Rilke wrote to a friend of this solitude which is filled with the presence of God: 'Love your solitude and bear the pain which it has caused you ... For those that are near you are far, you say, and this shows that distance begins to grow around you. And when your nearness is far, then your distance is already among the stars and very great; be glad of your growing, into which you can take no one else with you, and be good to those who remain behind.'[12]

The daily bread, referred to by Jesus in his prayer, speaks to many of the companionship, strength and consolation which comes during these later years from a sharing in the Eucharist. Here they find their own brokenness caught up within the broken bread, their weakness strengthened and their needs supplied. It is here, too, that in thanksgiving and communion they are drawn into the gift of Jesus to his Father, given that all the world might live. The Eucharist sums up for them and brings to reality once more the paradox that life comes forth from death.

The mystery of the Trinity also becomes more central in the lives of many older people. It has a special relevance for those struggling with loneliness and isolation, or the pain of incapacity and dependence. It is in the shared life and love of the community of the Godhead that they come to find their true home and happiness. There they learn the meaning of selfless giving and of reaching out to others. Their prayer becomes other-centred. As Madeleine Sophie Barat wrote to a long cherished friend: 'It is getting late for us. The sun of our life is on the decline. When it grows low on the horizon and is ready to slip away, its fires deepen and it throws a stronger, richer light. May it be the same for us.' This radiating of God's love becomes the focal point of Christian ageing.

The challenge for the elderly as they reach this deep union with God is to trust that their coming to integrity can be the most fruitful time of life. For it is in ageing graciously that they become a source of inspiration and of love for all creation. It is they who through concern and prayer can help stem the tide of destruction which threatens this beautiful beleaguered world, and truly celebrate the preciousness of life.

It is perhaps the mature aged, rather than the young, who can become for us the prophets of our time, witnessing to a present pregnant with possibilities and pointing to a future filled with hope.

Notes

Chapter 1 Life's afternoon

1 Carl G. Jung — *Modern Man in Search of a Soul,* trans. W.S. Dell & Cary F. Baynes, Harcourt, Brace, Jovanovich, New York, 1933, p.107.
2 ibid., — p.106.
3 ibid., — p.108.
4 Thomas Merton, — quoted in Raymond Studzinski, *Spiritual Direction and Mid-life Development,* Loyola University Press, Chicago, 1985, p.14.

Chapter 2 Exploring universal patterns

1 Carl G. Jung, — *Collected Works,* ed. Sir Herbert Read *et al.* trans. R.F.C. Hull, 2nd ed. rev. Bollingen Series XVI, Princeton University Press, Princeton, New Jersey, 1970, p.41.
2 Carl G. Jung, — *C.G. Jung: Psychological Reflections,* ed. Jolande Jacobi, Routledge & Kegan Paul, London, 1971, p.138.
3 Carl G. Jung, — *The Portable Jung,* ed. Joseph Campbell, The Viking Press, New York, 1971, p.60.
4 Carl G. Jung, — *C.G. Jung: Psychological Reflections,* p.42.
5 Carl G. Jung, — *The Portable Jung,* p.61.
6 ibid., — p.66.
7 Carl G. Jung, — *C.G. Jung: Psychological Reflections,* p.39.
8 John Welch, — *Spiritual Pilgrims: Carl Jung and Teresa of Avila,* Paulist Press, New York, 1982, p.90.
9 Carl G. Jung, — *Collected Works VII,* p.171.
10 Erik H. Erikson, — *Childhood and Society,* W.W. Norton & Co., New York, 1963, p.251.
11 ibid., — p.246.
12 Carol Gilligan — *In a Different Voice,* Harvard University Press, Massachusetts, 1982, p.160.
13 ibid., — p.163.
14 Erik H. Erikson, et al., — Vital Involvement in Old Age, W.W. Norton & Co., New York, 1963, p.251.
15 ibid., — p.55
16 Carol Gilligan — op.cit., p.12.

17 Nancy Chodorow, *The Reproduction of Mothering*, University of California Press, Berkeley, 1978, p.167.
18 Janet Lever, 'Sex Differences in the Games Children Play', *Social Problems 23*, 1976.
19 Jean Baker Miller, *Towards a New Psychology of Women*, Beacon Press, Boston, 1976.
20 James W. Fowler, *Becoming Adult, Becoming Christian*, Harper & Row, San Francisco, 1984, p.45.
21 Carol Gilligan, op.cit., p.73.
22 ibid., p.171.
23 ibid., p.23.
24 Daniel J. Levinson, et al., *The Seasons of a Man's Life*, Alfred A. Knopf, New York, 1978, p.324.
25 W. Shakespeare, *As You Like It*, Act 2:Sc.7.
26 Daniel B. Leavitt, *A Faith for the Middle Years*, The Alban Institute Inc., Washington, 1982, p.5.
27 Daniel J. Levinson, et al., op.cit., p.39.
28 Carl G. Jung, *Modern Man in Search of a Soul*, p.109.
29 Daniel J. Levinson, et al., op.cit., pp.243, 242.
30 Erik H. Erikson, et al., op.cit., p.51.

Chapter 3 Adult crises or transitions

1 Dante Alighieri, 'The Inferno' in the *Divine Comedy*.
2 Erik H. Erikson, *Identity, Youth and Crisis*, W.W. Norton & Co. Inc., New York, 1968, p.163.
3 Evelyn E. & James D. Whitehead, *Christian Life Patterns*, Doubleday & Company, Inc., New York, p.50.
4 ibid., p.58.
5 William B. Yeats, 'Circus Animals' Desertion' in *The New Oxford Book of English Verse*, ed. Helen Gardner, Clarendon Press, Oxford, 1972, p.831.
6 Gerald O'Collins, 'The Second Journey: An Epilogue' in *The Australasian Catholic Record*, Vol. LXII No. 1, 1985, p.15.

Chapter 4 Mid-life developmental tasks

1 Carl G. Jung *Modern Man in Search of a Soul*, p.108.
2 Carl G. Jung, *Collected Works*, XVII.
3 Carl G. Jung, *Modern Man in Search of a Soul*, p.104.

4 J.A. Sanford, *Dreams and Healing*, Paulist Press, New York, 1978, p.90.
5 W.A. Miller, *Make Friends with Your Shadow*, Augsburg Publishing House, Minneapolis, 1981, p.83.
6 Carl G. Jung, *Collected Works*, XI:1, p.60.
7 Carl G. Jung, *Collected Works*, XXVII, p.198.
8 J. Welch, op.cit., p.166.
9 J.A. Sanford, *The Invisible Partners*, Paulist Press, New York, 1980, p.43.
10 Carl G. Jung, *The Portable Jung*, p.174.
11 I.C. De Castillejo, *Knowing Woman*, Harper & Row, New York, 1973, p.84.
12 Carl G. Jung, *Collected Works*, IX:1, p.29.
13 R. Tagore, *Gitanjali*, Macmillan, India, 1913, reprint 1974, p.42.
14 Daniel J. Levinson, op.cit., p.222.
15 A. De Saint-Exupéry *The Little Prince*, trans. Katherine Woods, Piccolo Books in assoc. with Heinemann, London, 1974, p.72.
16 T.S. Eliot, 'East Coker' in *Four Quartets*, Faber & Faber, London, 1944, p.31.
17 Daniel J. Levinson, op.cit., p.241.
18 J. Brewi & A. Brennan, *Mid-Life Directions*, Paulist Press, New York, 1985, p.136.
19 G.E. Vaillant, *Adaptation to Life*, Little, Brown & Co., Boston, 1977, p.309.

Chapter 5 The generative person

1 Bernice L. Neugarten, 'Adult Personality: Towards a Psychology of the Life Cycle' in *Middle Age & Aging*, ed. Bernice Neugarten, University of Chicago Press, Chicago, 1968, pp.139, 141.
2 Erik H. Erikson, et al., op.cit., p.37.
3 Erik H. Erikson, *Childhood and Society*, p.267.
4 James W. Fowler, op.cit., p.26.
5 ibid., p.27.
6 Erik H. Erikson, et al., op.cit., p.35.
7 James W. Fowler, op.cit., p.28.
8 Erik H. Erikson, *Identity, Youth & Crisis*, p.139.
9 George E. Vaillant, op.cit., p.232.

10 Robert C. Peck, 'Psychological Developments in the Second Half of Life' in *Middle Age and Aging*, ed. Bernice Neugarten, p.89.
11 ibid., p.90.
12 Evelyn E. & James D. Whitehead op.cit., p.131.

Chapter 6 Stress and burnout

1 Peter Tyrer, *Stress*, Sheldon Press, London, 1980, p.5.
2 Michael D. Mitchell, *Consultant Burnout: The 1977 Annual Handbook for Group Facilitators*, eds. J.E. Jones & J.W. Pfeiffer, University Associates, La Jolla, 1977, p.143.
3 John A. Sanford, *Ministry Burnout*, Paulist Press, New York, 1982, p.106.

Chapter 7 Understanding anger

1 Hanna Arendt, quoted in *Seasons of Strength*, E. & J. Whitehead, Doubleday & Co. Inc., New York, 1984, p.125.
2 Charles Schwab, quoted in 'Perils of the Pleaser', Joseph L. Hart pub. in *Loneliness*, ed. James Madden, Affirmation Books, Massachusetts, 1977, p.52.
3 Anna A. Terruwe, & Conrad W. Baars, *Psychic Wholeness and Healing*, Alba House, New York, 1981, p.45.
4 Conrad W. Baars, *Feeling & Healing Your Emotions*, Lagos International, New Jersey, 1979, pp.149-150.
5 Margaret Brennan, 'Patriarchy: The Root of Alienation from the Earth?', in *Thomas Berry and the New Cosmology*, ed. Anne Lonergan & Caroline Richards, Twenty Third Publications, Connecticut, 1987, p.59.
6 Carolyn Osiek, *Beyond Anger*, Paulist Press, New York, 1986, p.15.
7 Dawn Brett, 'Apotheosis', unpublished poem quoted in *Wounded Women*, Linda Leonard, Shambhala, Boston, 1983, p.130.

Chapter 8 Development and integration of sexuality

1 William F. Kraft, *Sexual Dimensions of the Celibate Life*, Andrews and McMeel, Inc., Kansas City, 1979, p.36.
2 Jack Dominian, *The Growth of Love and Sex*, Darton, Longman & Todd, London, 1982, p.7.
3 Erik H. Erikson, *Childhood & Society*, p.263.

4 Michael E. Cavanagh,
'Psychosexual Development' in *Human Development*, Vol. 4, No. 3, 1983, p.16.
5 Erik H. Erikson, et al.,
op.cit., p.96.
6 Michael E. Cavanagh,
op.cit., p.23.
7 Yves E. Raguin, 'Chastity and Friendship' in *Supplement to the Way*, 19, 1973, p.114.
8 Gerald May, *Will and Spirit: A Contemplative Psychology*, Harper & Row, San Francisco, 1982, p.185.

Chapter 9 Menopause and the climacteric

1 Bernice L. Neugarten, et al.,
'Women's attitudes toward the Menopause' in *Middle Age and Aging*, ed. Bernice Neugarten, p.195.

Chapter 10 Towards a spirituality of mid-life

1 Brian Swimme, *The Universe is a Green Dragon*, Pear and Company, Santa Fe, New Mexico, 1984, p.118.
2 Thomas Berry, *Thomas Berry and the New Cosmology*, ed. Anne Lonergan & Caroline Richards, Twenty Third Publications, Connecticut, 1987, p.108.
3 Brian Swimme, op.cit., p.120.
4 Maria Boulding, *The Coming of God*, SPCK, London, 1982, p.86.
5 ibid., p.37.
6 Elizabeth Grantham, 'Unless the Seed ...', unpublished poem.
7 Henri Nouwen, *Reaching Out*, Doubleday & Company, New York, 1975, p.68.
8 Evelyn E. & James D. Whitehead,
op.cit., ch.6.
9 Rainer Maria Rilke, 'For Lotte Bielitz', *Poems 1906-1926*, trans. J.B. Leishman, 2nd ed. New Directions, Norfolk, Connecticut, 1957.

Chapter 11 The challenge of ageing

1 Robert N. Butler, 'The Facade of Chronological Age' in *Middle Age and Aging*, ed. Bernice Neugarten, p.235.
2 Erik H. Erikson, et al.,
op.cit., p.13.
3 ibid., p.215.
4 ibid., p.169.
5 Joan Erikson, from an article in the *New York Times*, 1986.

6 Erik H. Erikson, et al.,
op.cit., p.131.
7 ibid., p.55.
8 Erik H. Erikson, *Identity: Youth & Crisis*, p.139.
9 Robert Frost, *The Poetry of Robert Frost*, ed. Edward Latham, Holt, Rinehart & Winston Inc., 1969.
10 Carl G. Jung, *Modern Man in Search of a Soul*, p.108.
11 Eleanor Garner, unpublished lecture.
12 Elsie Harwood & K.L. Irvine,
'Psychological Significance of the University of Queensland Longitudinal Study of Aging,' presented at XIIIth Annual Conference of International Assoc. of Gerontology, New York, 1985.
13 Elsie Harwood, 'Mental Deterioration — Prevention,' paper presented at the Q.C.O.A. seminar, Griffith University, Queensland, 1986.
14 Alfons Deeken, *Growing Old And How to Cope With It*, Paulist Press, New York, 1972.
15 Margaret H. Huyck, *Growing Older*, Prentice-Hall Inc., New Jersey, 1974, p.77.
16 Eugene C. Bianchi, *Aging as a Spiritual Journey*, Crossroad, New York, 1982, p.221.

Chapter 12 Care of the ageing body

1 Maria Boulding, op.cit., p.181.
2 Madeleine Sophie Cooney,
RSCJ — A Journal of Reflection, Vol. VI, No. 1, Winter, 1985, p.28.

Chapter 13 Some emotional and mental disturbances

1 Henri J.M. Nouwen, *The Wounded Healer*, Doubleday & Co., New York, 1972, p.86.
2 Etty Hillesum, *Etty: A Diary 1941–43*, trans. by Arnold J. Pomerans, Trian Grafton Books, London, 1983, pp.234 & 259.
3 J. Grimley Evans, *Update*, May 22, 1987, p.22.
4 Francis Braceland, *Psychiatry, Ministry & Pastoral Counselling*, ed. A.W. Richard Sipe & Clarence J. Rowe, 2nd ed., Liturgical Press, Minnesota, 1984.
5 Bernice L. Neugarten, et al.,
'Personality and Patterns of Aging', in *Middle Age and Aging*, p.177.
6 ibid., p.173.
7 Brian Swimme, op.cit., p.120.

Chapter 14 Suffering and death

1 Rainer Maria Rilke, *Letters to a Young Poet*, trans. Herter Norton, W.W. Norton, New York, 1954, p.35.
2 F.W. Nietzsche, quoted in V. Frankl, *Man's Search for Meaning*, p.xvi.
3 Ian Crowe, *Out of the Darkness — A Depressive reaches for God*, Christian Media, West Australia, 1982, p.21.
4 Anonymous, quoted in Mary Craig, *Blessings*, Hodder & Stoughton Ltd., Great Britain, 1979, p.136.
5 Pierre d'Harcourt, 'The Real Enemy', quoted in *Blessings*, p.139.
6 Teilhard de Chardin, *Le Milieu Divin*, Collins, Great Britain, 1964, p.89.
7 Bernard J. Bush, 'All Creation Groans', in *Suffering*, ed. Richard Gilmartin, Mercantile Printing Co., Massachusetts, 1984, p.32.
8 C.S. Lewis *The Problem of Pain*, W. Collins & Sons, Glasgow, 1983, p.81.
9 John Paul II, 'Salvifici Doloris', St Paul Publications, N.S.W., 1984, p.55.
10 ibid., p.56.
11 Martin Israel, *The Pain that Heals*, A.R. Mowbray & Co Ltd, London, 1983, p.91.
12 Antoine de Saint-Exupéry, op.cit., p.76.
13 Engelbert Schwarzbauer, *The Agony & Grandeur of Death*, trans. Matthew O'Connell, Liturgical Press, Minnesota, 1976, p.10.
14 George J. Dyer, 'Recent Developments in the Theology of Death' in *The Mystery of Suffering and Death*, ed. Michael Taylor, Alba House, New York, 1973, p.105.

Chapter 15 A spirituality of the later years

1 Teilhard de Chardin, op.cit., p.89.
2 Evelyn Whitehead, 'Religious Images of Aging', in *Aging and the Human Spirit*, ed. Carol Le Febre & Perry Le Febre, Exploration Press, Chicago, 1981, p.61.
3 Carl G. Jung, *Modern Man in Search of a Soul*, p.235.
4 Kathleen Fischer, *Winter Grace*, Paulist Press, New York, 1985, p.39.
5 Evelyn Whitehead, op.cit., p.64.
6 Jean Beaven Abernathy, *Old is Not a Four-letter Word*, Abington Press, Nashville T.N., 1975, p.113.

7 Brian Swimme, 'Science: a Partner in Creating the Vision', in *Thomas Berry and the New Cosmology*, op.cit., p.88.

8 Unknown, *Cloud of Unknowing*, ed. W. Johnston, Doubleday & Co. Inc., New York, 1973, p.53.

9 Basil Pennington, from a lecture on Centring Prayer.

10 Madeleine Cooney, op.cit., p.31.

11 Thomas Merton, in a letter to a friend.

12 Rainer Maria Rilke, op.cit., p.37.

SELECT BIBLIOGRAPHY

Anonymous, *The Cloud of Unknowing*, edited by W. Johnston, Image Books Doubleday & Co., New York, 1973.

Bianchi, Eugene C. *Aging as a Spiritual Journey*, Crossroads Publishing Co., New York, 1982.

_____, *On Growing Older*. Crossroads Publishing Co., New York, 1985.

Boulding, Maria. *The Coming of God*. SPCK, London, 1982.

Bouwsma, William. *Christian Adulthood*. Norton & Co., N.Y. 1978.

Brewi, Janice and Brennan, Anne. *Mid-Life*. Crossroads Publishing Co. New York, 1982.

_____, *Mid-Life Directions*. Paulist Press, New York, 1985.

Cannon, Noreen. 'Getting to Know Your Shadow'. *Human Development* Vol.6, No.4., 1985, pp.32-36.

Carroll, L. Patrick and Dyckman, Katherine M. *Chaos or Creation – Spirituality in Mid-Life*. Paulist Press, New York, 1986.

Cavanagh, Michael. 'The Impact of Psychosexual Growth on Marriage and Religious Life.' *Human Development* Vol.4, No. 3, 1983, pp.16-24.

Clift, Wallace B. *Jung and Christianity*. Dove Communications, Melbourne, 1983.

Conway, James. *Men in Midlife Crisis*. Cook Pub., Elgin, 1978.

de Castillejo, Irene C. *Knowing Woman*. Harper and Row, N.Y., 1974.

Deeken, Alfons. *Growing Old, And How To Cope With It*. Paulist Press, N.Y., 1972.

Dominian, Jack. *The Growth of Love and Sex*. Darton, Longman & Todd, London, 1982.

Erikson, Erik. *Childhood and Society*. Norton and Co., N.Y., 1965.

_____, *Identity: Youth and Crisis*. Norton and Co., N.Y., 1968.

Erikson, Erik, Erikson, Joan & Kivnick, Helen. *Vital Involvement in Old Age*. W.W. Norton & Co., N.Y., 1986.

Fischer, Kathleen. *Winter Grace*. Paulist Press, N.Y., 1985.

Fowler, James. *Becoming Adult, Becoming Christian*. Harper & Row. San Francisco, 1984.

Fox, Matthew, *Original Blessing*. Bear & Co., New Mexico, 1983.

_____, *Breakthrough: Meister Eckhart's Creation Spirituality in New Translation*. Doubleday an Co., N.Y., 1980.

_____, *A Spirituality Named Compassion*. Winston Press, Minneapolis. 1979.

Fried, Barbara, *The Middle-Age Crisis*. Harper and Row, N.Y., 1965.

Gallagher, C., Maloney, G., Rousseau, M. & Wilczak, P. *Embodied in Love*. Dove Communications, Melbourne, 1983.

Gidley, Isobelle & Richard Shears. *Alzheimers*. Allen & Unwin, Australia, 1987.

Gilligan, Carol. *In a Different Voice*. Harvard University Press, Cambridge, 1983.

Gilmartin, Richard (ed.) *Suffering*. House of Affirmation, M.A., 1984.

Gould, R.L. 'The Phases of Adult Life: A Study in Developmental Psychology.' *American Journal of Psychiatry*. Vol.129, November 1972, pp. 33-43.

Groeschel, Benedict J. *Spiritual Passages*. Crossroad, N.Y., 1984.

Huyck, Margaret H. *Growing Older*. Prentice-Hall, New Jersey, 1974.

Israel, Martin. *The Pain That Heals*. Mowbray, London, 1981.

John Paul II. *Salvifici Dolores*. St Paul's Publications, N.S.W., 1984.

Johnston, Robert. *He*. Harper and Row, New York, 1977.

_____, *She*. Harper and Row, New York, 1976.

_____, *We*. Harper and Row, New York, 1983.

Johnston, William. *The Inner Eye of Love*. Harper and Row, N.Y., 1978.

Joyce, Mary R. *How Can A Man And Woman Be Friends?* Liturgical Press, Collegeville, 1977.

Jung, Carl Gustav. *Collected Works*. Translated by R.F.C. Hull, Bollingen Series XX Vol.8, *The Structure and Dynamics of the Psyche*. Princeton University Press, Princeton, 1969.

_____, *Collected Works*. Translated by R.F.C. Hull. Bollingen Series XX Vol. 9i. *The Archetypes and the Collective Unconscious*. Princeton University Press, Princeton, 1959.

_____, *Collected Works*. Translated by R.F.C. Hull. Bollingen Series

XX Vol.9.i: *Aion: Researches into the Phenomenology of the Self.* Princeton University Press, Princeton, 1969.

_____, *Collected Works.* Translated by R.F.C. Hull. Bollingen Series XX Vol.17. *The Development of Personality* Princeton University Press, Princeton, 1969.

_____, *Collected Works.* Translated by R.F.C. Hull. Bollingen Series XX Vol.10.l. *Civilisation in Transition.* Princeton University Press, Princeton, 1969.

_____, *Modern Man in Search of a Soul.* Harvest Books, N.Y., 1933.

Kastenbaum, Robert. *Growing Old.* Thomas Nelson, Australia Pty. Ltd., Melbourne, 1979.

Keane, Philip S. *Sexual Morality.* Paulist Press, N.Y., 1977.

Kenel, Mary E. 'A Celibate's Sexuality and Intimacy.' *Human Development.* Vol.7. No.1., 1986.

Kraft, William. *Achieving Promises: A Spiritual Guide For The Transitions of Life.* Westminster Press, Philadelphia, 1981.

Kroll, Una. *Growing Older.* Fount Paperbacks, London, 1988.

Kubler-Ross, Elizabeth. *On Death and Dying.* Macmillan Publishing Co. N.Y., 1969.

Kushner, Harold S. *When Bad Things Happen To Good People.* Schocken Books, N.Y., 1981.

Lake, Alice. *Our Own Years.* Winston Press, Minnesota, 1979.

Leavitt, Daniel. *A Faith For The Middle Years.* The Alban Institute, Inc., Washington D.C., 1982.

Leonard, Linda. *The Wounded Woman: Healing the Father-Daughter Relationship.* Shambhala Pub., Boulder, 1982.

Lester, Andrew & Judith. *Understanding Aging Parents.* Westminster Press, Philadelphia, 1980.

Levinson, Daniel. *The Seasons of A Man's Life.* Alfred Kropf, N.Y., 1978.

Lewis, C.S. *The Problem of Pain.* Fount Paperbacks, Collins, Glasgow, 1940.

Lindbergh, Anne M. *Gift From The Sea.* Vintage Books, N.Y., 1955.

Linn, Dennis & Matt. *Healing Life's Hurts.* Paulist Press, N.Y., 1978.

Lonergan, Anne & Richards, Caroline (ed.) *Thomas Berry & The New Cosmology.* Twenty Third Publications, Connecticut, 1987.

May, Gerald. *Will And Spirit: A Contemplative Psychology.* Harper and Row, San Francisco, 1982.

Miller, Jean Baker. *Toward A New Psychology Of Women.* Beacon Press, Boston, 1976.

Miller, William A. *Make Friends With Your Shadow.* Augsburg Publishing House, Minneapolis, 1981.

Murphy, Sheila. *Mid-Life Wanderer.* Affirmation Books, M.A., 1983.

Nelson, James. *Embodiment.* Augsburg Pub., Minneapolis, 1978.

Neugarten, Bernice (ed.) *Middle Age And Aging.* University of Chicago Press, Chicago, 1968.

Nouwen, Henri & Gaffney, Walter. *Aging*. Image Books, Doubleday & Co. N.Y., 1976.
O'Collins, Gerald. *Second Journey*. Paulist Press, N.Y., 1978.
O'Connor, Peter. *Understanding The Mid-Life Crisis*. Sun Books, Melbourne, 1981.
Sanford, John. *Evil: The Shadow Side Of Reality*. Crossroad, N.Y., 1982.
——, *The Invisible Partners*. Paulist Press, N.Y., 1980.
——, *Ministry Burnout*. Paulist Press, N.Y., 1982.
Schmidt, J. *Praying Our Experiences*. St Mary's College Press, Winona, 1980.
Schwarzbauer, E. *The Agony and Grandeur of Death*. The Liturgical Press, Collegeville, Minnesota, 1976.
Sheehy, Gail. *Passages*. Dutton and Co., N.Y., 1976.
Snell, Brigitte. 'Contemplation, the Healing of Memories and Anger.' *The Way Supplement*. No.59. 1987.
Spencer, Anita. *Seasons: Women's Search for Self Through Life Stages*. Paulist Press, N.Y., 1982.
Storr, Anthony. *The Integrity Of The Personality*. Penguin Books, 1960.
——, *Jung*. Fontana, W. Collins & Sons, London, 1973.
Studzinski, Raymond. *Spiritual Direction & Midlife Development*. Loyola, Chicago, 1985.
Swimme, Brian. *The Universe Is a Green Dragon*. Bear & Company, New Mexico, 1984.
Taylor, Michael (ed.) *The Mystery Of Suffering And Death*. Alba House, N.Y., 1973.
Tyrer, Peter. *Stress*. Sheldon Press, London, 1980.
Ulanov, Ann Belford. *Receiving Woman: Studies in the Psychology and Theology of the Feminine*. Westminster Press, Philadelphia, 1981.
Vaillant, George E. *Adaptation To Life*. Little, Brown & Co., Boston, 1977.
Westberg, Granger. *Good Grief*. Joint Board of Christian Education of Australia and New Zealand, Melbourne, 1966.
Whitehead, Evelyn & James. *Christian Life Patterns*. Doubleday, N.Y., 1979.
——, *Seasons Of Strength: New Visions of Adult Christian Maturing*. Doubleday, N.Y., 1984.
Wolff-Salin, Mary. *No Other Light: Points of Convergence in Psychology and Spirituality*. Crossroad, N.Y., 1986.
Zullo, James. 'The Crisis of Limits and Midlife Beginnings.' *Human Development*. Vol.3, No.1., 1982.

INDEX

EDUCATING PSYCHE

Bernie Neville

0 85924 777 5

'Bernie Neville shows us that the essence of education is becoming excited about ideas.'

Colin Wilson

Educating Psyche is a book about good teaching. It gives insights into teacher behaviour and educational goals and provides a most useful overview of alternative ways of seeing learning.

Educating Psyche is about the psyche — the whole mind — and calls on what we have learned from Jung, Freud, Coué, Assaglioli, Moreno, Erickson and other students of the mind, to tell us how we might go about creating a fully human education. Neville presents each of the different figures clearly, explaining their contribution briefly and in terms immediately useful to the classroom teacher.

Educating Psyche challenges teaching styles that are excessively narrow and promotes flexibility in teachers. The book looks at indirect learning, suggestion, trance, psychodrama, relaxation, autogenics, bio-feedback, visualisation, intuition, mind-control and meditation — more options than could be used in one year.

Bernard Neville's sensible approach and calm exposition will appeal to all those involved in education.

TOO OLD TO CHOOSE?

Social Justice for Older Australians

Anglican Social Responsibilities Commission
Edited by: Heidi M.E. Dixon

0 85924 829 1

The number of older people in Australia aged 65 years and over is expected to double in the next fifty years. This increase has major implications for both the Church and the wider community.

This report from the Anglican Social Responsibilities Commission thoroughly explores three major areas of concern:

- the value and dignity of older Australians and the contribution they make to community life.
- retirement income considerations for older Australians.
- housing options for older Australians.

The Social Responsibilities Commission of the Anglican Church has entered the political arena in support of older Australians, many of whom are unable to plead their own cause. The Commission speaks to the community at large in the name of the Church itself, calling for a greater sensitivity among its members towards those who are old.

WOMANHOOD

Anna Holmes

0 85924 709 0

Womanhood will appeal to women of all ages with its fresh approach to the study of women's health. Rather than concentrate on one single aspect of a woman's well-being, *Womanhood* considers all areas of a woman's life. Anna Holmes conveys a highly sensible and natural message: that good health is a balance. In this way *Womanhood* differs from many contemporary texts on women's health as it recognises the spiritual, social and emotional aspects in a woman's life as well as the physical.

Womanhood offers insight into coping with disease, highlights the contributing factors to physical and emotional health and suggests available resources. *Womanhood* delivers a message of hope in its proposal that each person can make use of the resources they have in order to live happily. Problems that lead to a sense of powerlessness are dealt with while practical knowledge and advice ensures that every woman has the opportunity to develop a whole and healthy life.

FACING CANCER

Searching for Solutions

Liz Byrski

0 85924 601 9

People with cancer and their families are faced with a bewildering choice of therapies. These range from the simple herbal remedies of ancient times to the latest sophisticated discoveries of modern medical science. They span diet, medication, physical treatment, meditation, imagery, lifestyle changes, psychological and spiritual philosophies.

How can people make decisions about appropriate treatment and sort fact from fiction and prejudice from honest concern?

This book provides an information base from which individuals may choose to make further investigations of some options or to discard them.

THROUGH A WOMAN'S EYES

Encounters With Jesus

Christine Burke

0 85924 826 7

After meeting Jesus we see life with new eyes. For two thousand years people have shared this experience. Each age returns with fresh questions to the original stories, seeking the light Jesus' life might shed on their particular situation.

Recent study has reclaimed the role of women in passing on these stories as apostles, preachers and leaders of communities.

Through A Woman's Eyes shares some of these insights with a wider public. The author and the artist hope that readers might discover, alone and with others, the excitement of the 'Good News' and recognise their role in keeping alive Jesus' message.

A new energy is released when women as well as men are encouraged to be leaders in our community and boundaries set by particular customs are questioned by the freedom of Jesus.

IN STILLNESS CONQUER FEAR

Overcoming Anxiety through Meditation

Pauline McKinnon

0 85924 782 1

Fear — we all encounter it from time to time. Many are crippled by fears that never leave their side. For most this need not be so.

Agoraphobia — the fear of leaving the safety of home — affects more people than one would imagine. After years of failing to overcome her own agoraphobia, Pauline McKinnon found a solution in meditative relaxation. *In Stillness Conquer Fear* is the record of her discoveries.

Already thousands of readers have found its insights are as illuminating as they are practical.

In this revised edition, three chapters are added to her original book detailing the practice of meditation and its benefits for agoraphobia sufferers. Those familiar with Pauline McKinnon's writing will find this expanded version valuable and confirming.